# conceivable

# conceivable

## The Insider's Guide to IVF

Jheni Osman

GREEN TREE
LONDON • OXFORD • NEW YORK • NEW DELHI • SYDNEY

Typeset in Minion Pro by Deanta Global Publishing Services, Chennai, India
Printed and bound in Great Britain by CPI Group (UK) Ltd., Croydon, CR0 4YY

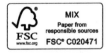

# Contents

# Foreword

The field of reproduction and fertility treatment is developing rapidly. Techniques and the technology used are evolving at pace, and more people than ever seek specialist help in order to conceive.

In my years working as a gynaecologist and fertility specialist, I've watched how fertility treatments have evolved and I've been at the front line of new developments, offering patients the opportunity to enhance their prospects of having a child.

We recognise the profound effect the work we do can have in changing people's lives, how important it is for them to have families, and we take this seriously. As such, helping in the creation of a life is one of the greatest things to be involved in. I am often humbled by the experience. Of course, in my job there are difficult moments, such as when patients are unable to have the longed-for baby in which they have invested so much time, financial resources, energy and emotion.

In my role as head of the Bristol Centre for Reproductive Medicine (BCRM), I see many patients who ask where they can find out more about IVF and all that it entails. There's never been one book to guide them through the whole process, while explaining the science behind what's involved, and providing insight from patients and experts alike. Until now. This practical, warm, all-you-need-to-know science-based guide will help you to understand the process and pressures of IVF, and help make what can be a very challenging journey easier – and, hopefully, successful.

*Dr Valentine Akande, MBBS PhD MRCOG, Consultant*
*Gynaecologist, Fertility Specialist and Reproductive Surgeon*

# Introduction

I f you're reading this book because you're struggling to have a baby, and you're thinking of having IVF, you're not alone. In the UK, around 3.5 million couples are finding it difficult to conceive, and thousands of fertility treatment cycles take place every year (over 74,000 cycles in 2018).

It's estimated that, to date, $25bn (£19.10bn) has been generated globally from fertility services such as IVF and egg freezing. It's no wonder it's big business. There are already more than 6 million people who were born via IVF. And one study even estimated that by the year 2100, 3 per cent of the world's population may exist because of assisted reproductive technologies – either they'll have been born through IVF themselves or be a descendant of an IVF baby.*

IVF, ICSI, IUI, glue, hatching, scratch... the fertility world can be overwhelming with its bizarre-sounding jargon and different acronyms for different treatments. If you're feeling bamboozled by stats, are suffering from information overload and weighed down by pharma-babble, then I hope this book will help you cut through the journal jargon and well-meaning blogs. And say goodbye to the lonely middle-of-the-night sessions browsing countless fertility sites, and lunch hours surreptitiously sifting through confusing, even contradictory, clinic leaflets. This guide is your IVF companion.

*Unless otherwise stated, throughout the book, for ease of reference, I refer collectively to fertility treatments such as IVF and ICSI as IVF.

1

Jessica Hepburn, author of *The Pursuit of Motherhood, 21 Miles* and founder of Fertility Fest, says…

'People do not understand that around three-quarters of all treatment cycles fail. I think we need to get that out there so people are prepared that they might need to go through more than one round of treatment or it might not even work. There is not enough information about the success rates, and what decisions you might need to make and when.'

First up, chapter 1 looks at some of the main reasons why people struggle to conceive, and what can be done to improve the chances of fertility treatment working. Chapter 2 explains the science behind how IVF and other treatments like ICSI work. Chapter 3 is a guide to choosing a clinic, discussing the costs involved in undergoing treatment, and which 'add-ons' might be worth investing in and which aren't. Chapter 4 discusses egg, sperm and embryo donation, and chapter 5 looks at what's involved in freezing them – and when might be best to do so. Chapter 6 explores the difficult subject of how to cope when IVF doesn't work. And, finally, chapter 7 runs through cutting-edge fertility treatments and what's on the horizon. Throughout the book there is help and guidance to help you handle challenging moments, as well as advice on where to look for further information. Depending on what stage you're at, you may want to skip forward to a particular chapter that's relevant to you. Maybe you've been trying for a while and want to know what the science says about improving your odds (start at chapter 1). Or maybe you're just considering freezing your eggs or sperm, in which case go straight to chapter 5 (although you'll probably find it useful to read the other chapters at some point to get an idea of the whole process of IVF and what will be involved once you thaw an egg or sperm). Or maybe you're interested in what your future options might be (turn to chapter 7).

Every person going through fertility treatment will have a different story and, hence, a slightly different journey. While writing this book, I've tried to cover as many different experiences and demographics as possible to give you a comprehensive picture of what fertility treatment involves, whether you're a solo parent, same-sex couple, heterosexual couple, egg or sperm donor... But I haven't been able to cover every single base, so I hope you can excuse me for that – otherwise this book would be way too long!

Trying to keep up with the latest fertility research or make sense of a new study on a fertility forum can lead to confusion about what to ask for at your clinic, or what treatments will have the best results. I've investigated all the latest research and, using my experience as a science journalist, extracted the studies that I feel are comprehensive and backed up by other research. Of course, in any particular piece of research, it's always worth bearing in mind that one factor that seems to have a beneficial effect may be influenced by other positive lifestyle changes that are not taken into account by that specific study. And there will always be one study that contradicts the vast body of evidence and grabs the tabloid headlines. But my job is to seek out the truth as best I can – even if in reality there is no black-and-white answer but current research points to shades of grey.

As well as sharing my own IVF story, I've spoken to numerous friends, colleagues and associates about their journeys. I've also interviewed many experts from different fields involved in the fertility industry and been advised by Dr Valentine Akande, Medical Director at the Bristol Centre for Reproductive Medicine, and Dr Chandra Kailasam, Consultant at the London Women's Clinic. All their expertise and insights will hopefully be useful, so that you can choose the right path for you.

'It's been such a journey. My husband and I had a very close relationship anyway – we've known each other since we were young – but going through this process has definitely ▶

brought us even closer. I know people who've split up because going through IVF and failing to get pregnant has just been too much pressure on their relationship. It did the opposite for us.' PIP

## CREATING FAMILIES

'Going through IVF actually brought my wife and I closer together. We were definitely in it together and there for each other.' ANON

Over the decades, fertility research and treatments have come on in leaps and bounds, with success rates that IVF pioneers Robert Edwards and Patrick Steptoe could only have dreamed of when they started carrying out the procedure back in the late 1970s. In the early days, success rates were less than 10 per cent per cycle of treatment. These days, according to the Human Fertilisation and Embryology Authority (HFEA), in 2018 the average birth rate per embryo transferred for all IVF patients was 23 per cent, and for women under 35 it was even higher, at 31 per cent.

Louise Brown – the first IVF baby – is now in her 40s. When I interviewed her for a Radio 4 *Costing the Earth* programme about fertility, I asked what she felt had been IVF's greatest achievement. She said: 'Creating families. Seeing the smiles on people's faces when they're finally pregnant, they carry and give birth.'

I'm immensely grateful to Louise's parents, and to Edwards and Steptoe, and the thousands of researchers around the world. My husband Max and I have ourselves had quite a journey, going through a few cycles of IVF and dealing with a failed round, yet we now have two children, both conceived through IVF – and we feel incredibly lucky.

It's this feeling of being lucky and grateful that has spurred me to write this book, to help others ensure that they give themselves the best chance of having a family if they want one. For whatever reason you've picked up this book, I hope it helps you on your IVF journey.

## What is IVF?

In vitro fertilisation (IVF) literally means fertilisation between an egg and a sperm outside of the human body. *In vitro* is just the Latin for 'in glass'. Standard IVF usually involves having to take various drugs for a number of weeks to control the woman's natural menstrual cycle and boost egg production. The eggs are then extracted from the ovaries, fertilised with the partner's (or donor's) sperm in a glass Petri dish, and then the embryo is inserted (transferred) into the womb (uterus).

## What is ICSI?

Intracytoplasmic sperm injection (ICSI) works exactly the same as IVF, except during fertilisation the sperm is injected directly into the egg, as opposed to them just being put in the same Petri dish.

## QUICK REVISION: SEXUAL REPRODUCTION

Before getting into the detailed nitty-gritty of what different fertility treatments involve, it's worth having a quick reminder of that cringeworthy biology lesson we all sat through at school.

When girls are born, their **ovaries** hold millions of fluid-filled sacs called **follicles**, which each contain an immature **egg**. This stash is all she'll ever have. A baby has about five to seven million eggs, but by puberty most of her remaining eggs will have deteriorated and been reabsorbed. Less than half a million will remain. Indeed, throughout her life she will constantly lose eggs, even if she's on the contraceptive pill. Once she reaches sexual maturity, around once a month an area in the brain known as the hypothalamus signals the pituitary gland to release **follicle-stimulating hormone (FSH)**, prompting some follicles to mature. The pituitary gland then releases **luteinising hormone (LH)**, which stimulates the most developed follicle to release an egg – this is called **ovulation**. The egg is only ripe for **fertilisation** for 12 to 24 hours after ovulation.

In contrast to women, who are born with all their eggs, men constantly produce fresh **sperm** every day throughout their lives. Sperm take up to three months to fully mature, as they travel from the **testes** to a narrow coiled tube on the outer surface of each testis where sperm are stored and mature, known as the **epididymis**. Tadpole-shaped, the sperm use their tails to propel themselves along, while the head contains the genetic material.

After **ejaculation**, there are all sorts of obstacles for sperm to get around in their race to the egg – from the acidic environment in the **vagina** to the female immune system, which could see the sperm as a 'foreign invader'. Considering they have to overcome all these hurdles in a relatively brief window of opportunity, it's just as well evolution has ensured that each male ejaculation releases millions and millions of sperm – anywhere between 40 million and 1.2 billion of them, all jostling for first place in the vagina, which is a hostile environment to hang around in.

Sperm are well prepped for the acidic environment of the vagina, though – after ejaculation, a protective **gel** forms around each one. Also, during ovulation, the vagina drops its defences, becoming less acidic, and the **cervical mucus** thins to let the sperm pass through.

Once inside the **uterus** (womb), the sperm get a helping hand in the form of a sort of wave machine – contractions push them along the **fallopian tubes**. The athletic ones can survive there for up to five days.

Similarly, the egg gets helped along the fallopian tube. The finger-like end of the tube is covered in adhesive tiny hairs, known as **cilia**. As the end sweeps over the ovary, it picks up the released egg, before the cilia and muscular contractions shunt it down the tube, ready for its speed date with sperm.

Of the millions of sperm that started the arduous journey, usually only one will make it over the threshold and into the inner sanctuary of the egg. The egg is surrounded by a membrane known as the **zona pellucida**. This contains sperm receptors – sites specifically designed for human sperm to latch on to. It's not necessarily the first sperm to arrive at the egg that gets the gold medal, but the one to penetrate the zona pellucida. Once one sperm has passed through, the membrane becomes impenetrable to any other. (Although in very rare cases two sperm have been

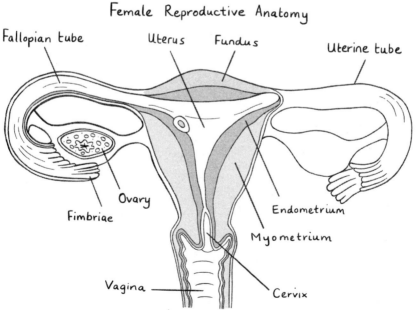

Female Reproductive Anatomy

known to penetrate and fertilise the egg simultaneously, producing semi-identical twins.)

The fertilised single-celled **embryo** is known as a **zygote**. Fertilisation kick-starts a series of cell divisions (**mitosis**). After three to four days, the embryo is a 16-cell mass called a **morula**. Then, within five to six days, it becomes a multi-cellular **blastocyst**, made up of several hundred cells. At this stage it is ready to implant itself in the uterus lining – the endometrium.

## CHAPTER 1

# Why can't we conceive?

## Reasons why you might be struggling to have a baby

While 80–90 per cent of couples trying for a baby will get pregnant within one year, you may be in the 10–20 per cent who struggle. Everybody's body is different. Throughout our lives, we all have various health issues to contend with – and for some of us that is fertility. Yet the one-size-fits-all fertility recommendations dished up by the media aren't helpful.

About a quarter of people that seek fertility treatment suffer from 'unexplained infertility', where there is no clear reason for not being able to conceive. But often there is an explanation, and there are specialist fertility consultants who will be able to identify the issue and work with you to try to resolve it. So, if you've been trying to conceive for over a year, then your first port of call should be your GP, who will be able to offer advice (*see* page 10). But if you still don't have any success after two years, then your GP should refer you on to a specialist fertility clinic (although if you're a woman and 36 and over, or a man and 40 and over, then your GP should refer you before the two-year mark).

## GP advice

If you've been struggling to conceive, chat to your doctor, who will make some of the suggestions below about ways you can improve your chances of getting pregnant naturally...

- **Have sex every two to three days.** To give yourself the best chance of conceiving, you should have sex roughly every other day during the fertile phase of the menstrual cycle – which is typically between day 10 and day 18 if you have a regular cycle. If you don't have regular periods, it's probably worth having sex through much of your cycle, so you don't miss the window of opportunity. But obviously there needs to be a healthy balance between your sex life and your overall well-being – and not feeling too much pressure to be having sex constantly or to get the timing exactly right.

**Ovulation** is when an egg is released from one of your ovaries. After release, it survives for about 12 to 24 hours and so has to be fertilised by the sperm within this window of time. Sperm can live for up to five days inside a woman's body. So if you have sex in the days leading up to ovulation, the sperm will have had time to travel up the fallopian tubes and be ready for when the egg is released.

If you have regular periods, ovulation occurs around 10 to 16 days before your period starts. You may know when you're ovulating as you might secrete some clear or white mucus from your vagina – it looks a bit like runny egg white. Your body temperature might rise a little too, but doctors advise against taking your temperature – it's unreliable. Instead, you could try using an ovulation predictor kit, which measures hormone levels in your urine.

- **Don't smoke.** Smoking dramatically affects egg and sperm quality (see page 35).
- **Don't drink too much.** Drinking excessive amounts of alcohol affects egg and sperm quality (see page 34).
- **Stay fit – but don't over-exercise.** Your BMI should ideally lie somewhere between 19kg/m² and 30kg/m² (see page 28).

Body mass index (BMI) is calculated using your height and weight to work out if your weight is healthy.

As well, men should...

- **Avoid taking anabolic steroids**. Steroids, such as those taken for muscle building in the gym, can affect sperm quality (*see* page 50).
- **Wear baggy boxers.** Tight pants, hot baths, saunas, and laptops on laps can all heat up your testicles and affect sperm production (*see* page 45).

And general points...

- **Avoid getting pregnant when visiting certain countries.** Research has shown that exposure to Zika virus during pregnancy can cause birth defects. So if you're travelling to places with Zika virus, use contraception to avoid getting pregnant there and for three months after leaving that country.
- **Get medical advice if you've been unwell.** Some viral infections, such as coronaviruses, can cause a high fever.

  As of June 2020, current evidence suggests that, while it is likely that COVID-19 can pass from mother to baby, the virus does not cause problems with a baby's development or cause miscarriage. No other coronavirus has been found to cause foetal abnormalities, and routine scans in Asia suggest that this is probably also the case for COVID-19. Evidence also suggests that there is no greater risk that pregnant women who develop COVID-19 will become more seriously ill than other healthy adults. But, it's not possible to be absolutely certain.

  There have been a few reports that some women who have been seriously unwell with COVID-19 have given birth to premature babies – but it's currently unclear whether this is because medical staff recommended the babies were born early. In all known cases, newborns that have developed coronavirus very soon after birth remain well.

  All this information is drawn from the limited evidence from COVID-19 combined with evidence from similar viral illnesses. For the latest information visit the website of the Royal College of Obstetricians and Gynaecologists (RCOG).

# WHY SOME WOMEN MAY STRUGGLE TO CONCEIVE

If you're struggling to conceive, there could be a problem with your reproductive anatomy – your ovaries, fallopian tubes, uterus (womb) or cervix. In this section you'll find some questions to consider. If you think you may suffer from any of the conditions outlined in this section such as those below, it's worth having a chat with your GP, who can arrange for various tests.

## Tests

A surgery, clinic or hospital can carry out various tests to check for any issues with your reproductive anatomy, as recommended by your doctor. Depending on your situation, these might include:

- Blood test – identifies viruses and bacteria, such as the sexually transmitted infection chlamydia (see page 16), and assesses hormone levels that could affect ovulation, such as follicle-stimulating hormone (FSH), luteinising hormone (LH) and prolactin, as well as levels of anti-Müllerian hormone (AMH), which gives an indication of the ability of the ovaries to produce eggs (ovarian reserve).
- Ultrasound scan – analyses ovaries and uterus, or tracks the development of a follicle.
- Hysterosalpingogram (HSG) – checks fallopian tubes using an X-ray.
- HyCoSy (Hysterosalpingo Contrast Sonography) – an alternative to HSG, this checks fallopian tubes using contrast gel under ultrasound guidance.
- Laparoscopy – checks fallopian tubes by an operation under general anaesthetic, where a thin tube with a light and camera on the end is inserted through a small incision in the abdomen.
- Hysteroscopy – checks for fibroids or polyps by examining the inside of the uterus via a thin tube with a light and camera on the end, which is inserted via the vagina and cervix.
- Biopsy – analysis of the endometrium by taking a tissue sample from it, usually under local anaesthetic. However, this is not a routine test unless the doctor suspects some issue. ▶

An ultrasound scan showed that although I didn't have premature ovarian insufficiency (see explanation of POI below), my 'ovarian reserve' was low. Basically, my ovaries weren't producing many follicles with eggs in. This is more common over the age of 40, but when Max and I first started trying to get pregnant I was 35.

## BIOLOGICAL FACTORS

## Do you have regular periods?

The most common reasons for not ovulating are if a woman suffers from polycystic ovaries or premature ovarian insufficiency (POI). Thyroid problems (an underactive or overactive thyroid) are occasionally to blame for lack of ovulation.

## Premature ovarian insufficiency (POI)

This is a loss of ovarian function before the age of 40, where the ovaries stop producing normal levels of oestrogen and may not produce eggs. It's also known as 'primary ovarian failure'.

## Polycystic ovary syndrome (PCOS)

PCOS is when a woman has ovaries with a large number of follicles that don't release eggs. It is known to run in families and is the most common form of female infertility – around one in five women worldwide are thought to suffer from it, but over half of them don't have any symptoms. Those who do have symptoms may have irregular or non-existent periods, acne, be overweight or grow excessive amounts of hair – usually on the face, chest, back or bottom.

Although until recently the causes of PCOS have been unknown, research now indicates that it may be linked with a hormonal imbalance before birth. A study in 2018 suggested that excessive levels of anti-Müllerian hormone (AMH) may affect the development of a female foetus, who could then suffer from PCOS in later life.

**Metformin** tablets can be taken two to three times a day to help manage polycystic ovary syndrome.

## Thyroid problems

Your thyroid gland in your neck makes two hormones that are secreted into the blood: thyroxine (T4) and triiodothyronine (T3), which are vital to keep all the cells in your body working normally. If you have an underactive thyroid gland (hypothyroidism), it does not produce enough hormones, while an overactive thyroid (hyperthyroidism or thyrotoxicosis) produces too much of the hormones, both of which interfere with ovulation.

## Have you had any surgery?

If a woman has had abdominal or pelvic surgery the fallopian tubes can be damaged or scarred, which can block them. Similarly, cervical surgery can scar the area or shorten the neck of the womb. (Too much or extra sticky cervical mucus can also be a problem – preventing sperm getting through.)

### Dr Chandra says…

'If the endometrium is not optimal, then it does not matter what kind of embryo you put in. It's like putting a seed in the soil in the garden – the seed may be fabulous, but if the soil is not good, it's never going to take.'

## Do you suffer from endometriosis?

Endometriosis occurs when tissue from the endometrium grows outside the uterus, damaging the ovaries or fallopian tubes. The condition can affect fertility, but exactly why isn't yet fully understood – it's thought it could be something to do with the damage to the ovaries or fallopian tubes. The condition can be painful, particularly during periods or sex. Other symptoms include chronic pelvic pain, nausea, constipation or diarrhoea, or blood in your urine during your period. An estimated 176 million women worldwide suffer from the condition, and it affects all ages. Your fallopian tubes can be checked and endometriosis identified in an ultrasound scan or laparoscopy (*see* page 12). It can be quite difficult to treat, but there has been some success using hormone medicines, or via surgery to cut away patches of endometriosis tissue. Talk to your doctor if you have any concerns.

### Dr Valentine says…

'Endometriosis is a big problem when it causes pelvic pain, scarring or blockage of the tubes, or when there's a cyst [a fluid-filled sac that develops on an ovary]. We see a lot of people with endometriosis who have no problem getting pregnant. There's no question endometriosis affects fertility, but not everybody who has endometriosis has subfertility. I prefer not to give patients' conditions names without a full explanation, because if one says, "You've got endometriosis", one just hears, "endometriosis" – most would have no concept about where they sit in the spectrum. It would just be like saying, "You live in a house", but it could be a hut or Buckingham Palace. They're both houses. But they're very different. The same thing, when people hear "polycystic ovaries". They think the worst. Actually, if you have polycystic ovaries but not the syndrome, it means you've got lots of eggs – and that can be a good thing.'

'After an early miscarriage, we found out my wife had endometriosis and ovarian cysts, which required surgery to remove the cysts. Following this, our consultant advised that we wait no more than six months of trying to conceive naturally due to the amount of scar tissue around the fallopian tubes. After no luck after six months, we embarked on IVF. We had a "light" IVF cycle (*see* page 95). We were told that as my wife was relatively young (31 at the time), there was a good chance of IVF working, so that gave us hope.' **VENKI**

## Do you have an STI?

Most of us would like to think 'of course not!' But the reality is that a surprising number of us do carry a sexually transmitted infection.

Chlamydia is the most common bacterial STI in the UK – especially prevalent in teenagers and young adults. In England in 2018, 49 per cent of all new STI diagnoses were for chlamydia. Passed on through unprotected sex, in women symptoms include a painful tummy, bleeding after sex or between periods, pain when peeing, or unusual discharge. The problem is that mild chlamydia often doesn't show any symptoms, so many people don't realise they've got it, but if untreated it can cause all sorts of long-term health problems – and, crucially, infertility. The disease affects both male and female fertility.

It is thought that chlamydia damages the tiny hairs in the fallopian tubes that help the egg travel from the ovaries to the uterus. This can cause scarring and eventually block the tubes. Treatment usually involves a course of antibiotics, but if the fallopian tubes are badly damaged by the disease, then consultants tend to recommend going straight to IVF. Although about 45 per cent of infertility caused by damage to the fallopian tubes *might* be attributable to chlamydia infection, the probability of tubal infertility in women who have had chlamydia is estimated to be only 1–4 per cent.

Gonorrhoea and mycoplasma also affect fertility.

## Jheni's story…

I remember receiving all my blood test results prior to embarking on IVF. Neither Max nor I had chlamydia, but I was surprised to see the STI down on the list as a potential reason for subfertility.

Dr Chandra explained: 'When I tell patients that their blood test for chlamydia is positive, the vast majority of them are very upset – because of the perceived stigma. I tell them: It doesn't mean you have chlamydia now, it's like a fingerprint – you might have been exposed to it 5, 10, 15, 20 years ago and your blood test continues to be positive.'

## Have you had cancer treatment?

One in two people in the UK will be diagnosed with some sort of cancer during their lifetime, and 9 per cent of these cancer cases affect people between the ages of 30 and 49. While cancer is more prevalent in the older population, many younger people get cancer – often in their crucial fertile years.

Chemotherapy drugs can cause temporary or permanent infertility. It all depends on your body and the dosage of drugs. When you're going through treatment, it's likely that your periods will become irregular or stop. In about a third of women, they will return to normal 6–12 months after your treatment is over. But if you're taking a high dose of drugs, they can sometimes cause irreversible damage to the ovaries, particularly if you're older and nearing the menopause. It's worth chatting to your doctor before undergoing any cancer treatment to be sure you're fully aware of all the facts, in case you want to, for example, freeze your eggs.

Dr Valentine says…

'If someone has a high ovarian reserve [lots of eggs] and goes through chemotherapy, their reserve will drop to normal, that's fine. But if someone starts with a normal reserve, chemotherapy will bring them down to low levels.'

## Are you taking or have you ever taken any recreational drugs?

Illegal drugs, such as marijuana or cocaine, can mess with ovulation and cause irregular periods.

Marijuana interferes with the secretion of luteinising hormone (LH), which normally triggers ovulation. Also, its active ingredient – tetrahydrocannabinol (THC) – slows down a fertilised egg as it passes through the fallopian tubes, so the embryo might not make it to the uterus in time to implant. Either it will break down and be ejected from the body, or it might implant in the tube, resulting in what's known as an ectopic pregnancy. If you've been prescribed CBD oil for medical purposes, check that it doesn't contain THC.

## FEMALE LIFESTYLE AND ENVIRONMENTAL FACTORS THAT COULD AFFECT CONCEPTION

There are also lifestyle factors that can have an effect on conception, so they're worth considering if you want to improve your chances.

## Age

In many countries around the world there is a trend towards older mothers. Increased access to higher education, more opportunities for working women and improved contraception mean more of us are having children later in life.

A review in 2011 found that in the US the birth rate in women aged over 35 had increased by almost 60 per cent since 1980, whereas the birth rate for women aged between 20 to 34 had gone up by only 10 per cent.

This trend is also happening in Europe. In the UK, a 2018 report by the Office for National Statistics showed that pregnancies in under-18s had fallen by more than 50 per cent in less than 30 years, and conception rates had dropped among women in their late 20s and 30s for the first time in a decade. And yet the one group that saw a rise in pregnancy rates from 2015 to 2016 were the over-40s. In large part this is due to fertility treatments. Over the last few decades, the average IVF patient age has increased from 33.5 in 1991 to 35.3 in 2018 (and for donor insemination from 32 to 34.5). This is probably due to improved treatment techniques. Yet age is the biggest factor

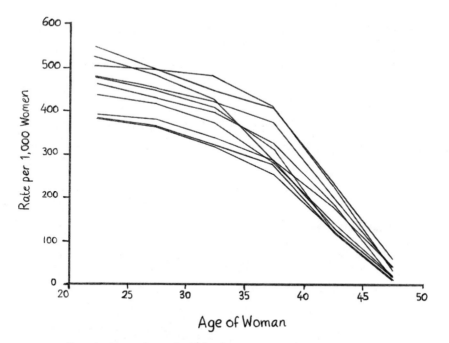

Graph shows how fertility declines in women according to age. Source: ACOG, published in 2014.

affecting fertility – and the female biological clock stops ticking earlier in women than in men.

Normally, female fertility decreases gradually through our 20s, slowing down around 32 years of age, and then rapidly declining from the age of 37. The Human Fertilisation and Embryology Authority (HFEA – the government's independent regulator that oversees fertility treatment and research) states that 95 per cent of women aged 35 and under who have regular sex will get pregnant within three years of trying, but by the age of 38 only 75 per cent will.

Jheni's story…

Before starting IVF myself, I didn't realise a woman's fertility declines so early in life. One of my best friends was surprised by this: 'Jhen, how didn't you know this! You studied biology with me!' In my defence, I did know it decreased – I just didn't realise how soon and how rapidly. I had other things on my mind in my early 30s and, arrogantly, didn't think that it would be a problem for healthy-living me. Yes, I was naive! But I'm not alone.

A study of university students to find out whether they are aware of this declining fertility showed that less than half of them knew what age the decrease kicks in.

Dr Valentine says…

'Age is the most important factor that affects fertility. It's simply that the younger egg is more robust. Between the ages of 18 and 31 women are most fertile. Between 31 and 41 fertility decreases, becoming more profound at 36, 37. Then ▶

statistically at 41 it's the end of fertility. It's at that age where the challenges mount significantly. It doesn't mean one can't get pregnant; however, if one embarks on trying to conceive at 41 years of age, over 50 per cent will not be successful at having a baby without help. Many women over 45 with a child would have had egg donation treatment. Whereas men can have children in their 80s – although over 40 their fertility starts to decline, but there's not this drop-off cliff. As such, with regards to age and fertility, I say to patients that your chances today are better than tomorrow, and your chances yesterday were better than they are today.'

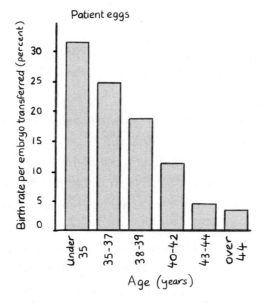

Graph shows birth rates per embryo transferred by age bands, 2019. Source: HFEA.

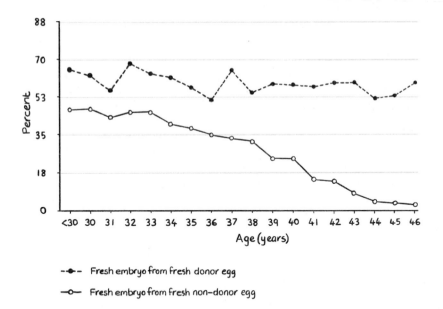

Fresh embryo from fresh donor egg

Fresh embryo from fresh non-donor egg

Graph shows percentage of transfers using fresh embryos from donor or patient eggs that resulted in live births by age of woman, 2018.

## Stress

How many times have you heard: 'Just relax and it'll happen? You're too stressed, just chill out.' Not helpful *at all*. Smiling through gritted teeth, I bet you've felt like shouting back, it's really hard to 'chill out' when you've just heard the 'wonderful news' that Lauren on reception is due with her third child, and last night you had to coax Mr Partner upstairs again when you'd both rather just be watching the rest of a box set on the sofa. Or maybe you've remortgaged the house to go through your third cycle, your stomach feels like a punchbag from injecting all the drugs and now you're in the horrible two-week waiting zone until you can take a pregnancy test. Thanks, well-meaning friend (or simply annoying colleague), but I have a right to feel stressed.

However empathetic someone is, until they experience what it's like not to be able to have a child, they won't understand how harrowing it can be. Indeed, some people find being unable to have children due to infertility as being comparable to grieving over a death.

Often stress is blamed for someone not being able to get pregnant. But research is conflicting as to whether this is the case or not.

One study led by researchers at the Boston University School of Public Health (BUSPH), which was published in 2018, found higher levels of stress were associated with lower odds of conception for women who were trying to get pregnant naturally (but not for men), although the researchers did point out that this could be because the stressed couples were having sex less frequently.

But work by Professor Jacky Boivin, an expert in developmental psychology at the University of Cardiff, suggests the opposite. Back in 2011, Boivin reviewed 14 studies where 3583 infertile women had been assessed for anxiety and stress before they began treatment. Her results showed that stress didn't affect the chances of becoming pregnant.

'Our findings show that there is no reason for them to fret any more that any difficulties they are facing may prevent them from becoming pregnant,' says Boivin. 'They can at least relax about that.'

This sounds like good news. But there is a catch. Boivin's research suggests that although stress itself doesn't affect fertility, your actions in response to feeling stressed might do. For example, when we're stressed we tend not to eat well – not eating enough or over-eating. Maybe you're tempted to have just one cigarette, or your partner starts smoking again. Or maybe you're so fed up of 'doing it' that you just want some time off from having scheduled sex.

'When you're stressed, you do things that are really bad for your fertility,' says Boivin. 'But, importantly, you tend to stop trying to conceive. Either you're not having sex as often as you would be if you weren't stressed, or you decide to drop out of treatment. Of course, if you're not trying, then you're not going to be able to achieve pregnancy.'

Other research looked at whether stress affects the chances of getting pregnant when specifically going through fertility treatment.

Back in 2005, a Swedish study of 166 women found no evidence that psychological stress had any influence on whether fertility treatment worked or not. And, in 2018, researchers at Stony Brook University in New York looked at 20 different studies, involving more than 4300 women. Their findings also cast doubt on the idea that stress inhibits the success of fertility treatment.

> 'When we started IVF I wasn't in the right frame of mind. I was frustrated and angry that we had to do IVF. When I look back now, no wonder it didn't work – I was so stressed and in such a foul place.' **ALANA**

All of these conflicting studies mean it is difficult to be definite about whether stress does have a role to play in success rates for fertility treatment. I guess the main thing is it can't hurt to be as relaxed as possible going through IVF (see below for 'stress busters') and to be aware of not slipping into bad habits to compensate when feeling stressed.

## Stress busters

If you're feeling overwhelmed and anxious that this could be affecting your chances of conceiving, here are some ways you can feel calm and in control of your IVF journey.

- **Think positive.** Easy to say, yet not so easy to do. But research at Staffordshire University found that people who view a demanding situation as *challenging* perform a lot better than those who see it as *threatening*. Of course, you can't think yourself pregnant and you need to be realistic (the average birth rate for women of all ages using their own eggs is 23 per cent). But staying positive could ensure you don't slip into bad habits, such as indulging in something that could affect your chances of success.
- **Talk to someone.** You may want to keep the fact that you're going through IVF to yourself, but it can help to have at least

▶

one confidante to discuss how you're feeling. In general, research has shown that engaging with others buffers stress and gives you perspective on challenges you may be facing.

- **Get moving.** Exercise is known to reduce stress, as shown by loads of different studies. The Mayo Clinic in the US reckons that this is the case because it causes 'runner's high', raising levels of endorphins – the brain's feel-good neurotransmitters. It also makes the brain focus on just the movement, taking your mind off things. But don't overdo it – excessive exercise can affect fertility (*see* page 30).

- **Escape outdoors.** Even if you live in a city, you can give yourself a good dose of nature every so often. Many studies have shown that being outdoors in a green space (whether that's the countryside or just your garden or allotment) reduces things like cortisol levels, heart rate and blood pressure.

- **Eat well.** Aside from adopting a Mediterranean diet (*see* page 33), consuming prebiotics helps to boost the growth of good bacteria in your gut. Research has shown that eating foods high in prebiotics, such as garlic, leeks, onions and bananas, helps extend the key sleep phase known as REM, helping you to recover from stress. This is backed up by other research, which found that eating lots of fruit and veg each day lowers the risk of stress.

## Complementary therapies

Some IVF patients try complementary therapies, like acupuncture and reflexology, in the hope that it'll improve their chances of getting pregnant. But such therapies do split opinion. While practitioners may claim that their treatment can improve fertility and/or increase IVF success rates, medical professionals that I spoke to were reticent about whether it really helped, saying there was little scientific evidence for such claims, and it was important to look at where funding came from for any studies on the benefits of complementary therapies. Others said it might well be down to the placebo effect, where the actual treatment has no physiological benefit in itself, but positive results are seen because a patient believes the treatment is good for them.

So it's worth bearing all this in mind if you're considering any complementary therapies. However, such treatments can be very relaxing and enjoyable, so you may just want to give it a go anyway as a way of spoiling yourself through the challenging journey of IVF.

This was the case for me. Reflexology involves applying pressure to specific parts of the body, usually on the feet, but also on the hands and even the ears. The theory is that putting pressure on these 'reflex points' instigates change or healing in a related organ elsewhere in the body.

Even though I was sceptical of the science of how reflexology supposedly worked, I decided to try it as I thought it might make me feel good and help me cope with going through IVF. And it did. I had a wonderful therapist, Sarah, who became a bit of a confidante and counsellor. I enjoyed the sessions immensely, which combined a lovely relaxing treatment with a good natter about how I was feeling. Crucially, Sarah was not a family member or friend, but someone completely separate from my personal life, so it was easy to talk to her without having to worry about any other agendas. And Sarah ensured that she worked around what the clinic was doing, so during the down regulation phase of menstrual cycle suppression (see page 66), she was careful not to stimulate my system too much. Who knows if reflexology made any difference as to whether IVF worked for me or not? (I had reflexology for each of the three cycles of IVF that I went through, and IVF worked two out of three times.) But after each session I certainly felt nicely chilled and ready for the next stage.

If you're thinking of having a complementary therapy, try to find a therapist with experience of treating people with fertility problems and make sure they are a qualified practitioner, who is registered with the relevant regulatory body. Ensure that the therapist does not do anything that will cause harm or counteract the work of the clinic, such as working against the action of certain drugs. And it's worth budgeting for treatments in advance, as the cost of weekly sessions can quickly add up.

## Q&A

Professor Edzard Ernst, Emeritus Professor at the University of Exeter, and co-author of *Trick or Treatment: The Undeniable Facts about Alternative Medicine*, discusses what the science says about complementary therapies with regard to fertility treatments...

Q. What does scientific evidence show about complementary therapies in relation to IVF?

A. Three of the most recent reviews tell us that no treatment in addition to the primary treatment has been shown to be definitively advantageous; there are no significant benefits of acupuncture to improve outcomes of IVF and the currently available literature does not provide sufficient evidence that acupuncture improves IVF clinical pregnancy rate. Another study [published in 2018] concluded that 'among women undergoing IVF, administration of acupuncture v sham acupuncture [using a placebo] at the time of ovarian stimulation and embryo transfer resulted in no significant difference in live birth rates. These findings do not support the use of acupuncture to improve the rate of live births among women undergoing IVF.'

Q. What about studies that suggest there may be some benefit?

A. Many acupuncture studies come from China, and there is plenty of evidence to show that these are notoriously unreliable or even falsified.

Q. Why in your opinion is there relatively little research into the effect of alternative therapies on fertility treatment?

A. Researchers tend to focus on promising targets and funders give money for plausible projects. Alternative therapies do not fall into this category.

Q. If complementary therapies make the patient feel good, then what's the harm in having a treatment?
A. The harm is diverse and significant: the therapists take money and that harms the clients' bank accounts; by pretending they have an effective treatment, the therapists delay or prevent an effective therapy being used; by making consumers believe in implausible concepts, therapists undermine rational thinking;

contrary to widespread belief, alternative therapies are not free of side effects – for instance, acupuncture causes adverse effects in around 10 per cent of all cases; in addition, it also causes serious complications such as infections, injuries to vital organs (pneumothorax) and even deaths.

## Weight

Us women are always beating ourselves up about our weight. But, sadly, and I hate to have to say this, if you're underweight or overweight you could find it more difficult to conceive.

Research shows that you're more likely to suffer from things like irregular periods if you're overweight. It's because overweight women have higher levels of the hormone leptin, which is produced in fatty tissue. Leptin is thought to regulate fat storage in the body, but also to affect reproductive hormones.

Other studies have found that, during fertility treatment, overweight women respond less well to drugs that improve or regulate ovulation, meaning fewer eggs are produced. Fertilisation rates are also lower and embryos are not as high quality in women – even younger women – who are overweight.

The National Institute for Health and Care Excellence (NICE) guidelines recommend that BMI should ideally lie in the range 19–30 before starting treatment. Indeed, most NHS Clinical Commissioning Groups (CCG) won't treat women with a BMI below 18.5 (Scotland) or 19 (England) and above 30. (The NHS classifies an adult as a healthy weight if they have a BMI of 18.5 to 24.9, overweight if they have a BMI of 25 to 29.9, and obese if they have a BMI of over 30.)

One study showed that women with a BMI over 27 were three times less likely to conceive because they didn't ovulate, compared to women in the healthier weight range. And, even if a woman does ovulate, another study showed that the chances of conceiving within a year go down by around 4 per cent for every unit of BMI above 29.

Also, there is a higher risk of losing the baby in early pregnancy. Indeed, the chance of a live birth through IVF drops by 9 per cent in women who are overweight and 20 per cent in obese women.

So losing weight could improve your odds. But some experts feel BMI shouldn't be a deciding factor as to whether a couple can try for a baby or not. 'If someone has a BMI of 40, they're extremely unlikely to get back to 25 or under,' says Robert Norman, Professor of Reproductive and Periconceptual Medicine at the University of Adelaide in Australia. 'Denying them any treatment based on BMI is increasingly looking untenable. In New Zealand, for instance, if you've got a BMI of 32, you can't get public funding. In Australia, it's recommended that no one with a BMI of 35 should receive fertility treatment. But I believe women and their partners need choices, provided they have the full information to make a clear decision and know that if they're overweight, their chances of getting pregnant are lower, their chances of miscarriage are higher, and their chances of pregnancy complications are higher. If they have sincerely tried to lose weight (there has to be a track record of having tried), I don't think we as medical people should withhold reasonable treatment from them. Otherwise you're condemning a lot of overweight people, saying: "Well, because you're overweight, we're never going to do anything to help you have children".'

Dr Valentine says...

'If a woman's BMI is over 35, there's a higher risk of miscarriage. So, it's not just about your ability to get pregnant, it's also about being able to maintain the pregnancy.'

Being underweight can be just as detrimental to fertility as being overweight. Less research has been carried out on this, but in one piece of research a doctor in Chicago analysed data from 2362 cycles of IVF involving women under the age of 40. Patients with a BMI between 14 and 18 had only a 34 per cent chance of getting pregnant, compared to those with a 'healthy weight' (a BMI between 19 and 28), who had a success rate of 50 per cent.

This seems to be the case the world over. 'Underweight is also a problem. I had one particular patient with a BMI of 17, who denied any eating disorder,' says Professor Norman. 'She went through 18 cycles without success. But when she put weight on and her BMI got up to 20, she became pregnant. She now has three children.'

## Exercise

As with many lifestyle choices, a moderate amount of activity is a good thing and experts would recommend you build some easy exercise into your day when you're trying to conceive. But excessive exercise has a detrimental effect on success.

In 2018, a meta-analysis (a study of studies), involving 3683 infertile couples in total, found that the women who were more active before undergoing treatment had slightly better success rates than those who weren't.

But research also shows that extreme training reduces fertility. This is certainly the case with female sportswomen, who are pushing their bodies to the limit.

Various studies suggest this is because the body may not have enough energy to support both hard workouts and getting pregnant. Extreme exercise can interfere with reproductive hormones, causing irregular or non-existent periods. One study of almost 3000 women revealed that frequent and hard physical exercise seems to reduce fertility in young women. Another study of 2232 women undergoing IVF found that cardiovascular exercise for four hours or more a week over the course of a year leading up to treatment reduced the chance of a live birth by 40 per cent and the embryo not implanting. The good news is that fertility seems to recover if training is reduced.

## Dr Valentine says…

'If you have a low BMI, you have a much lower chance [of getting pregnant], and there's a higher risk of miscarriage. That's why in some areas the NHS doesn't offer IVF treatment to women with a BMI under 19. There are people who run marathons and think it's healthy, but most are not designed to do that. It's a huge stress on the body. Some people might stop having periods. For example, some ballet dancers don't have periods at all, as it makes them have a thin [uterus] lining. In others, we find the micro-environment around the egg is affected. Their hormone responses are blunted. So then the quality of the eggs isn't good, and that translates into the quality of the embryo.

For example, I recall a patient was trying for three years, and was still having periods. She did three cycles of IVF treatment. Two didn't work, the embryos were suboptimal. The third cycle was much better because she gave up running marathons. Three months later, she got pregnant naturally.

It also depends on genes. But for anybody doing "excessive" exercise, I advise to tone it down. A lot of people don't realise that it takes four months to "recruit" an egg. An "insult" in the preceding four months prior to ovulation could actually have an effect on the quality of the eggs. That's why patients who, for example, smoke or run marathons [one habit not healthy, the other on the surface of it very healthy] would in both cases have to wait four months before starting the drugs.'

'Prior to our successful cycle, I significantly reduced the amount of exercise I was doing. Being active was a massive part of my life, so cutting this down was hard and, at times, quite depressing. We will probably never know if it was a contributing ▶

factor in the successful outcome, but it did mean I had more energy and took up Pilates, yoga and relaxation in place of sports, which I feel was a positive. I do think reducing the volume and intensity of exercise helped, and personally I would take the same approach if going through IVF again.' **SOPHIE**

'I think reducing extreme exercise did help a little, but it was a balancing act as exercise also helped reduce stress for my wife, so it was important to keep a balance.' **ED**

## Diet

What you eat obviously affects your weight, but you could be within the 'healthy weight' bracket yet have an unhealthy diet that affects your fertility.

There is a whole host of books out there on 'IVF diets' or ones to improve your fertility. Many are well-meaning and could be useful to take a look at. But the one book that is recommended by many in the scientific community is *The Fertility Diet* by Jorge Chavarro and Walter Willett – professors of Epidemiology and Nutrition at Harvard University, whose research examined in depth the effects of diet and other lifestyle changes on fertility among 18,000 women. For people trying to get pregnant naturally, the researchers suggest avoiding artery-clogging trans fats (from processed foods) and red meat, and instead eating 'good fats' such as nuts, seeds, and oily fish like salmon and sardines; adding in vegetable protein like beans, peas or tofu; choosing slow-releasing carbohydrates that are high in fibre, such as whole grains, as these control blood sugar level; ensuring you get plenty of iron from wholegrain cereals, spinach, beans, pumpkin, tomatoes and beets; and drinking whole milk – or even having a small dish of ice cream or full-fat yogurt every day. But it's important to note that these recommendations are aimed at those dealing with ovulation issues, as opposed to physical problems such as blocked fallopian tubes.

Other smaller studies have looked into diet for people going through IVF. And it seems that much the same foods are recommended.

A small study published in 2010 of 161 couples undergoing IVF at Erasmus University Medical Center in Rotterdam, the Netherlands, found that they were 40 per cent more likely to get pregnant if they ate a Mediterranean diet high in fish, fruit, veg, whole grains, pasta, rice and olive oil – and less red meat.

A more recent study from 2018 backs this up. An Assisted Conception Unit in Greece looked at the diets of women going through their first IVF treatment. Those that ate a Mediterranean diet were 65–68 per cent more likely to become pregnant than those who ate far less of the recommended foods. This was particularly pronounced in women younger than 35, while a Mediterranean diet didn't seem to affect the chances of women who were 35 or older – possibly because other factors, such as having fewer eggs, masked the effect of the diet. The researchers were keen to point out that their results couldn't automatically be extrapolated to women who are overweight, those being treated in clinics in other countries, or women trying to conceive naturally.

The reason a Mediterranean diet improves fertility could be due to its effect on the health of your eggs. Professor Norman and his team in Australia have researched how egg health is affected in animals fed a high-fat diet. 'When we looked at their eggs, they were severely damaged and didn't fertilise well. And the animals didn't produce healthy offspring – if they produced any at all. But by putting these animals back on to a low-fat diet and exercise, we were able to reverse it. So we would assume it would be the same in human eggs and that you can alter the quality of the egg in the way that you eat. That's probably how something like the

Mediterranean diet works. By having fatty acids that are less toxic to the egg.' (Certain fats are a key part of our diet, because they ensure our cells communicate with each other. The body can't make essential fatty acids, so we need to get them from foods such as fish, which is rich in omega-3.)

'So, if you're trying to get pregnant naturally, and you're a "normal" weight the professor continues, you're probably better off on a Mediterranean type diet of 1400–1600 calories a day, taking folic acid, doing adequate exercise, avoiding alcohol and reducing the amount of caffeine to no more than two or three cups a day. But if you want to have chocolate cake once a day, that's fine, as long as you're not taking very much else.'

## Caffeine

Caffeine often gets scrutinised when considering its effect on health. Professor Norman's suggestion of no more than two or three cups a day is supported by the most recent research, which shows there is little evidence that a moderate amount of caffeine has a detrimental effect. However, NICE does say: 'maternal caffeine consumption has adverse effects on the success rates of assisted reproduction procedures, including IVF treatment'. Obviously, this contradicts the recent research. The best option might be to cut out caffeine altogether, or just keep it to a minimum.

## Alcohol

The risks of alcohol on a developing foetus are well known, so most women trying to conceive will have cut right back on how much they drink. But many different pieces of research also show that even moderate amounts can affect whether IVF works or not. The reason seems to be that alcohol affects egg quality.

A 2017 study on 221 couples undergoing fertility treatment found that consuming one extra drink a day (compared to those who had one less in the weeks before treatment) resulted in 13 per cent fewer eggs being retrieved, almost three times less chance of conceiving and over two times higher risk of miscarriage.

Another study of 4729 IVF cycles found live birth rates were reduced for women who consumed four or more drinks a week while going through treatment, compared with those who drank fewer than four. And the stats were even worse for heterosexual couples if both partners had more than four drinks a week.

The science behind why this is the case is as yet unknown. But it could be that, as excessive drinking increases the levels of certain hormones, eggs may mature abnormally and the endometrium not be as receptive to implantation.

NICE says: 'the consumption of more than 1 unit of alcohol per day reduces the effectiveness of assisted reproduction procedures.'

## Smoking

Smoking also drastically reduces your chances of getting pregnant. Even if you don't smoke, but your partner does, your chances are lower, as you're exposed to secondary smoke in the air. Indeed, a paper published in 2018 found that non-smokers' fertility was as badly affected by excessive exposure to second-hand smoke as if they smoked themselves.

Various pieces of research have revealed why this is the case. A Dutch study back in 2005 found that smoking adds the equivalent of 10 years to a 20-year-old woman's reproductive age, while more recent research found that smoking may advance the time of menopause by up to four years. Also, smoking can affect the fertility of a developing foetus. A number of studies have found a link between mothers that smoke during pregnancy and reduced sperm counts in their male offspring.

And for those going through IVF, smoking has been found to affect treatment. Smokers require nearly twice the number of cycles to conceive compared to non-smokers, while a paper published in 2018 revealed smoking reduces the thickness of the endometrium in women going through IVF. And a Spanish/Portuguese study back in 2006 found that women who did not smoke, or those that smoked fewer than 10 cigarettes a day, were 50 per cent more likely to have a baby.

Stats like these make a very clear case for quitting cigarettes. Of course, this can be easier said than done. But the NHS won't fund IVF for anyone who smokes.

Dr Valentine says…

'The key thing you'll notice about people who smoke and have babies is that they tend to be young. You don't see an old person smoking who has a baby, do you? The reason is that the eggs of a young person are more resilient and robust, and the embryos are more likely to repair.'

## Vaping

While smoking electronic cigarettes (vaping) has been promoted as being safer than smoking tobacco, the flavoured solutions may contain harmful contaminants like nitrosamines and diethylene glycol. A study published in 2019 suggested that vaping may harm fertility in young women, because of its effect in mice. After exposure to e-cigarette vapour, embryo implantation was lower and the onset of pregnancy delayed in female mice. Female offspring exposed to the vapour also failed to gain as much weight.

It's still early days and not much research has been done on the overall health effects of smoking e-cigarettes, but it may be worth considering this research if you've switched from smoking tobacco to vaping.

## Pollutants

Where you live or work could affect your chances of getting pregnant, as air pollution has been found to affect fertility.

A 2018 study revealed that embryo implantation and live birth success rates were lower for women going through IVF who lived close to major roads. Another study, in 2010, showed a similar result – lower success rates after IVF if exposed to air pollutants, particularly nitrogen dioxide, which is emitted when fuels are burned such as in a petrol or diesel engine. And research published in 2014 on women in Barcelona, Spain, showed an increase of just 3.5 micrograms of polluting particles per cubic metre caused fertility to decline by 13 per cent.

No one quite knows why air pollution affects fertility. It could be down to inflammation caused by pollutants, or the fact that particles contain tiny traces of heavy metals and so disrupt our reproductive hormones. All we do know is that our bodies are very sensitive.

Dr Valentine says…

'When building work was being done next to our clinic, we had to have all the windows sealed [to protect against pollutants, such as dust], install extra air filters and use air-quality monitors. We know of two clinics who got very poor pregnancy rates because of building works nearby. Embryos are so sensitive.'

## WHY SOME MEN MAY STRUGGLE TO CONCEIVE

For around half of all heterosexual couples who are struggling to conceive, the cause of the problem is related to sperm.

'Male fertility has been under-studied and under-talked about over the decades,' said Allan Pacey, Professor of Andrology at the

Department of Oncology and Metabolism, University of Sheffield, when I interviewed him for the Radio 4 series *Costing the Earth*. 'Men are quite reticent about coming forward. Science has been quite reticent about studying it. And funders have been reticent about funding it. The difficulty we have is that, while it's very easy to work out who the mother is because the woman gets pregnant, it's less easy to work out who the father is. Most population statistics about fertility are recorded in terms of the number of births per woman, rather than the number of paternities per man.

'There is a broad relationship between the number of sperm a man has and the quality of those sperm – how well they're swimming, how well they're put together, how well the DNA is packaged in the sperm head.

'There are scientists that say sperm quality has declined. I'm still a little on the fence about whether that is a real effect or not. It's very hard to unpick when that started or by how much that has changed. We're only in the foothills of fully understanding how male infertility may have changed or may be changing.'

There have been some studies trying to investigate whether male fertility is declining. The results from one study, published by an international team in 2017, certainly suggested men may be becoming less virile than they used to be. The results showed a 52 per cent drop in sperm concentration, and a 59 per cent decline in total sperm count, among men from North America, Europe, Australia and New Zealand, in the past 40 years. This suggests that sperm counts in the West have more than halved in the last few decades, and are dropping by an average of 1.4 per cent every year.

'Male factor infertility doesn't get spoken about very much. I'm pleased to say that's slowly changing, but I guess we're our own worst enemy because, in general, men don't like to talk about these things.' RICHARD

## BIOLOGICAL FACTORS AFFECTING SPERM QUALITY AND FUNCTION

Conception success is affected by poor-quality sperm – for example, if they are bad swimmers. In some cases it's not clear why they're not good quality, but sometimes it's linked to:

### A structural problem

For example, if some of the reproductive anatomy is blocked or damaged by illness, injury or previous surgery, if the male had undescended testicles as a baby, or if he has a condition such as varicoceles, where the veins that drain the testicles become swollen.

### A hormone imbalance

This is caused by conditions such as hypogonadism, where the body does not produce enough testosterone, which impacts on fertility. This can be treated with medicines containing testosterone, such as gels or injections.

### A genetic condition

For example, men with Klinefelter syndrome have an extra X chromosome. (Chromosomes are the structures inside cells that carry genes and are mostly made of DNA. People normally have 23 pairs of chromosomes, including an X and Y in men, or two X chromosomes in women.) Klinefelter syndrome is one of the most common genetic conditions in the UK, affecting around one in 600 men. But many people (even those who have it) have never heard of it, as the symptoms (tallness, fatigue, less body hair and small testes) can be difficult to spot. Between 95 and 99 per cent of men with Klinefelter syndrome are infertile, because they do not produce enough sperm.

## A genital infection

The STI chlamydia genetically damages the sperm by causing more than three times the normal level of DNA fragmentation – in other words, the DNA is broken apart. If the infection spreads to the testicles and epididymis (tubes that carry sperm from the testicles), they can become swollen and painful, which is known as epididymitis.

'The sperm quality of men who have an infection, such as chlamydia, is lower than it should be. But when you give the appropriate antibiotics, the sperm quality recovers,' says Professor Pacey. 'So a general piece of advice for anybody planning to start a family is simply to go and get yourself checked out. Often chlamydia doesn't have any symptoms, so you don't know that you have it.'

In terms of other STIs, gonorrhoea can affect fertility in the same way as chlamydia. Mycoplasma and herpes may also affect fertility, but research is minimal.

There are home kits that you can buy to test your sperm, but they just give a quick assessment of sperm count (and quality). Most don't identify other factors, so you might want to get a semen analysis done at a clinic.

Dr Valentine says…

'It's not a very peaceful analogy, but imagine you have an army of millions equipped with horses, lining up against a smaller army of thousands using motorised vehicles, it's very clear the latter would win. The smaller army, well equipped, will be more effective than a huge army with less sophisticated equipment. It's the same with sperm – quality over quantity.'

## Semen analysis

If you're struggling to conceive, it might be worth taking a semen analysis to see if there's an issue with your fertility. This basically involves masturbating into a special pot, which is then sent off to a lab. You can get the pot from your GP or from a fertility clinic, depending on who arranges for the test. The sample can be done at home and then dropped off at your GP or the clinic, or it can be carried out at the clinic in a private room. The results are usually available within a week. The standard semen analysis is quite detailed and will check your sperm for the following:

- **Sperm count.** According to the World Health Organization (WHO), the average man will ejaculate a volume of around 1.5 millilitres of semen – roughly three teaspoonfuls. A low sperm count, known as oligozoospermia, is where a man has fewer than 15 million sperm per millilitre of semen.
- **Morphology.** This refers to the shape of the sperm. A 'normal' sperm cell basically looks a bit like a miniature tadpole with a head and long tail. If a sperm cell is an 'abnormal' shape, it'll be harder for it to move and fertilise an egg. In the average man, three out of 10 sperm cells have abnormalities. The WHO recommends that at least 4 per cent of the semen sample should have a normal shape.
- **Motility.** This refers to how well the sperm move. If they don't move well, they will struggle to swim to the egg to fertilise it. On average, 40 per cent of sperm are bad swimmers. Yet the WHO recommends for fertility purposes that at least 32 per cent or more have good motility.
- **Presence of anti-sperm antibodies.** When the body's immune system launches an attack on sperm, antibodies may cause them to stick together (agglutinate) or hinder their ability to swim or fertilise. These antibodies are fairly rare but can occur if the man has had a bad groin injury, an operation on his reproductive anatomy, or a reversal of 'the snip' (vasectomy).
- **Concentration of white blood cells.** If there's an unusually high number of white blood cells in the semen, they weaken the

sperm and can damage the genetic material. This condition is known as pyospermia or leukocytospermia.

If you do decide to go ahead with IVF, you might go through something called 'sperm recovery', where the sperm are put through a challenge to see how many can be used for insemination. A good analogy is like taking soldiers and trying to select the SAS. So from 250 million sperm, 10 million might be selected.

## LIFESTYLE AND ENVIRONMENTAL FACTORS THAT COULD AFFECT MALE FERTILITY

### Age

When rock star Mick Jagger became a father to his eighth child at the age of 73, he beat the odds. Sure, men don't go through the menopause like women, but they do also have a biological clock, even if we don't hear it ticking as loudly.

Research has shown that as a man gets older his sperm quality declines, it takes longer to conceive and miscarriage rates for his partner increase. There is also an increased risk in various health conditions and birth defects for any children that are conceived. (The same goes for older mothers.)

Male fertility starts to decline around the age of 40 to 45, because the number and quality of sperm produced decreases. A study found that couples where the man is 45 or over are five times more likely to take more than a year to conceive compared to men in their 20s.

Another study found that women with partners aged 35 and older were 27 per cent more likely to experience a miscarriage than those with partners who were 25 or younger. This was irrespective of the woman's age.

Despite all this, many men are leaving it longer before they start trying for a family. A review in 2011 found that in the US the fertility rate for men in their 30s had increased by 21 per cent over the previous three decades, while for men aged 40 and over the rate had increased almost 30 per cent. This contrasted starkly with the fertility rate in men under 30, decreasing by 15 per cent. Another study, published in 2017, which looked at over 168 million births in the US, found that the average paternal age had risen from 27.4 to 30.9 years old over the previous 40 years. This increase occurred in all races and ethnicities and across all states and demographics but was particularly pronounced in men that went to university. And similar trends have been noted in the UK and other European countries.

The inevitable consequence of all this is that age-related male infertility is now a problem worldwide.

## Weight

All the evidence points to the fact that male fertility is affected by obesity – when someone has a body mass index (BMI) of over 30. In a 2015 review of 30 different studies, which looked at a total of 115,158 men, those who were obese were more likely to experience infertility, because more of their sperm were abnormally shaped or the DNA was fragmented. It also found that IVF was less likely to work using obese men's sperm and, even if it did result in a pregnancy, there was a 10 per cent higher risk that the foetus wouldn't survive, even if the mother wasn't obese.

An earlier study in 2014 revealed that fertility was probably lower because of a combination of factors: hormone issues, sexual dysfunction and other health conditions linked to obesity, like type 2 diabetes and sleep apnoea – both of which are connected with lower testosterone levels and erectile problems. The study estimated that carrying an extra 10kg of weight lowered male fertility by 10 per cent.

## Diet

As is the case with women, men can also benefit from a Mediterranean diet. Research has found that eating foods such as fish, poultry, whole grains, fruits, vegetables and nuts improves semen quality. One study focused in particular on nuts. A group of men who ate around a couple of handfuls of mixed almonds, hazelnuts and walnuts a day for 14 weeks had a higher sperm count and more mobile sperm than the non-nut-eating group.

## Exercise

Moderate exercise seems to be good for male fertility. But as with women and exercise, too much of a good thing can be detrimental.

A study back in 2009 found that men who exercised at least three times a week for an hour, generally had higher quality sperm (in terms of numbers, concentration and shape) than those who did more frequent and rigorous exercise. But too intense an exercise regime created poorer quality sperm, so elite athletes were the worst off.

This was backed up by a review in 2017 of the current research. It also showed that intense physical activity may affect quality – increasing the number of abnormally shaped sperm and reducing semen concentration, as well as the number of mobile sperm.

In recent years there has been a lot of discussion as to whether cycling affects male fertility, the idea being that the pressure from sitting on the saddle isn't good for the testes. Back in 2014, a study at University College London looked at the cycling habits of 5282 men, ranging from commuters to amateur racers, who were doing roughly four to eight hours in the saddle a week. The researchers couldn't find a link between cycling and infertility. One of the authors pointed out that modern-day saddles are better designed so that there's a lot less pressure on testes than there once was.

But a more recent study in 2018, which followed men undergoing 16 weeks of low to intensive cycling training, found that the exercise may have affected their fertility. This is also supported by some older studies.

So, while a short commute to work probably isn't a bad thing – particularly considering the other health benefits associated with cycling, which may improve fertility – it seems excessive training for amateur or pro cyclists *could* be detrimental.

> 'Round three of IVF my wife and I went on a massive health kick. I got really into fitness and yoga. And I did lots of research about zinc supplements, the best vitamins to take etc. After round three failed we kind of gave up hope and relaxed our health kick somewhat. Maybe this was the key. Or maybe it was just the right embryo.' **NICKY**

## Temperature

The testes sit in a scrotal sac outside the body, as they need to be a couple of degrees Celsius cooler than body temperature in order for sperm to develop inside. We've all seen the headlines – wear baggy boxers, don't put your laptop on your lap, avoid hot baths… Is there any truth to these suggestions?

The theory is that the extra heat generated from a laptop, hot bath, or tight underwear (which pulls your testicles up against the warmth of your body) affects sperm production. Indeed, research suggests that excessive exposure to heat can kill off germ cells (the cells that become gametes – male sperm or female eggs), damage sperm DNA and affect sperm shape.

A 2018 study at Harvard of 656 men found that those who wore boxer shorts had a 17 per cent higher sperm count, 25 per cent higher sperm concentration, and 33 per cent more swimming sperm than those who wore tighter briefs.

Research by Professor Allan Pacey and colleagues at Sheffield University also found this to be true. 'I was quite suspicious that tight underwear was a risk,' says Professor Pacey. 'But when we asked men what type of underwear they wore, we were able to see statistically that the men that wore tight underwear were about twice as likely to have poor sperm than men who wore looser boxer-type shorts.'

So, if you're trying to become a dad, research recommends switching your pants for a baggier option to improve your sperm quality. Although it's worth pointing out that changing your style of underwear on Friday won't improve your sperm by Monday, as it takes three months to produce sperm. Also avoid very hot baths and saunas, and be careful with laptops. There have been case histories with men who have actually burnt their penises by putting laptops on their laps, without wearing adequate clothing. This illustrates the dangers of heat on the underside of a laptop and the damage it can do.

### 'Cooking sperm'

Mobile phones often get a bad rap, with concerns spiralling over whether they affect our health. But research does back that up to a certain extent. A 2016 study found that mobiles could be 'cooking sperm'. More than 100 men who kept their phones in their pocket during the day were monitored for a year. The sperm of 47 per cent of them were 'quite seriously affected'. Likewise, a meta-analysis (study of 10 separate studies) found that exposure to electromagnetic radiation emitted by mobile phones was linked to sperm not moving or functioning as well as normal.

## Alcohol

If you're trying for a baby, giving up certain vices seems like a good call – and that includes excessive drinking. NICE guidelines recommend men drink no more than 4 units of alcohol a day. (A pint of normal strength beer is about 2 units and a small – 125 ml – glass of wine is about 1.5 units.) Experts think excessive alcohol consumption affects sperm quality and quantity, as well as reducing libido. The good news is that men constantly produce fresh sperm every day throughout their lives, so any negative effect can be rectified – although it's worth remembering that sperm take up to three months to fully mature.

When going through IVF, the NHS and most experts suggest that avoiding alcohol may improve the chances of having a baby. Indeed, back in 2009, Tony Rutherford, the then chairman of the British Fertility Society, said: 'If you are going to have IVF, my recommendation would be that it makes sense to avoid alcohol altogether, from three months beforehand.'

A 2009 study by doctors at Harvard Medical School on 2574 couples undergoing IVF found that the couples who shared a bottle of wine a week lowered their chances of getting pregnant by more than a quarter.

But more recent research suggests moderate amounts of alcohol may not be an issue. The problem is the lack of solid evidence, as participants are often also smokers and overweight or obese, so it's difficult to extract the effect of alcohol. A study of 8344 men that looked at the effect of drinking up to 8 units of alcohol per week, seven days before a semen analysis, didn't find any link between the two.

'In one of our studies, it was very interesting to find that drinking alcohol within guidelines isn't a major problem – although there's data to show that if you're a binge drinker that can be bad,' says Professor Pacey at Sheffield University.

Indeed, one study in 2018 even found that drinking a moderate amount of alcohol might boost male fertility – although the researchers admitted to not having an explanation for this. This surprising finding generated lots of headlines and could just be an example of that one study contradicting the vast body of evidence.

So, bearing all these different studies in mind, it seems that the odd drink isn't going to hurt, but excessive boozing or binge drinking should be avoided.

## Smoking

Unsurprisingly, research indicates that smoking is bad news for male fertility, since it damages sperm DNA, which affects sperm motility and shape, as well as sperm count.

In a 2010 study of 166 couples, if the man had smoked recently, only 7.8 per cent of the couples were successful in having a baby, compared to 21.1 per cent for non-smokers. Another study in 1998 of 498 couples found that if the male partner smoked, the chances of a successful pregnancy dropped by 2.4 per cent for every year older a male was. And a study in 2003 of 301 couples showed that paternal smoking was linked with significantly lower success rates for IVF (18 per cent versus 32 per cent in non-smokers) and ICSI (22 per cent versus 38 per cent in non-smokers).

Interestingly, a 2018 study showed that the sons of fathers who smoked while their partner was pregnant had half as many sperm as those with non-smoking fathers.

So all evidence points to quitting cigarettes if you're serious about starting a family. And it's worth knowing that the NHS won't fund IVF treatment for anyone who smokes.

## Vaping

As with women, there is some evidence that several electronic cigarette flavours may damage male fertility. But research into this field is still in its infancy.

## Drugs

Recreational drug use is fairly prevalent in the UK. NHS statistics show that in 2016–17, about 1 in 12 (8.5 per cent) adults between the

| The effect of alcohol, tobacco and recreational drugs on male reproduction | | |
|---|---|---|
| | Effect on hormones | Effect on sperm |
| Alcohol | ↑ LH & FSH levels<br>↓ testosterone levels | ↓ sperm shape<br>↓ sperm count and mobility<br>↓ sperm volume<br>↑ DNA damage |
| Tobacco | ↑/↓ LH & FSH levels<br>↑ testosterone levels | ↓ sperm shape<br>↓ sperm count and mobility<br>↑ DNA damage |
| Recreational drugs | Marijuana:<br>↓ LH levels<br>↑/↓ testosterone levels<br><br>Cocaine: ↑ LH levels<br><br>Opioids:<br>↓ GnRH secretion<br>↓ testosterone levels | ↓ sperm count and mobility<br>↑ DNA damage |

The effect of alcohol, tobacco and drugs on reproduction

ages of 16 and 59 in England and Wales had taken an illicit drug in the last year.

If you're trying for a baby, recreational drugs should be avoided, as a number of studies have found they impact male fertility. The studies showed that marijuana, anabolic steroids, cocaine and opioids all affected reproductive hormones or sperm in various ways, such as impairing their development, affecting their shape and how well they move, and reducing sperm counts.

'In one of our studies, men using cannabis were generally more likely to have misshapen sperm than men who didn't,' says Sheffield University's Professor Pacey. 'That is probably because of the compounds in cannabis, in a way that we don't yet understand. So if you're a cannabis user and you're trying to be a dad then it would be wise to stop that for several months before you try to start for a family.'

## Disease and medication

Male fertility is often affected by illness, whether that's something you're currently suffering from or an illness you've had in the past.

For example, just under half of all men who get mumps-related orchitis experience some shrinkage of their testicles and about 10 per cent have a drop in their sperm count – but it rarely causes infertility.

So, if you're trying for a family, it's worth getting any symptoms checked out by your GP, discussing your medical history, and seeking advice on medication.

Professor Pacey points out: 'Men who have transient infections, such as a fever for more than two weeks, can temporarily stop producing sperm. That's almost certainly because of "having heat" and being systemically unwell. One of the first things the body does when you're unwell is to shut down the production of sperm.'

---

### Medication that affects male fertility

There are many medications to avoid if you're trying to have a child, but here are a few key ones...

- Sulfasalazine. This anti-inflammatory is used to treat conditions like Crohn's disease and rheumatoid arthritis, but it has been found to lower sperm count. Stopping the medication, if possible, should return sperm numbers to normal levels.
- Anabolic steroids. Steroid misuse is becoming more common. Steroids are used to build up muscle and improve performance, but long-term use can reduce sperm count and how well they move.
- Chemotherapy. Chemo drugs can lower sperm counts and affect how they move, so men hoping to have a family are often advised to freeze sperm before undergoing chemotherapy.

---

## Environmental factors

In the last 60 to 70 years, scientists have known that something we're exposed to in our environment has been affecting male fertility, but they haven't had much luck in finding out exactly what that is. Some experts are blaming human-made substances, such as chemicals, pollutants and plastics.

- **Plastics:** When researchers first started realising that fertility was falling, it coincided with the discovery that there were more 'intersex' fish in rivers – where male fish were showing female characteristics. This was known to be caused by increased oestrogen exposure, and there was evidence that certain plastics were leaching chemicals that caused this. So, of course, scientists jumped to the conclusion that the two were linked.

  However, subsequent research has shown that this is too simplistic. For many years, Professor Richard Sharpe and colleagues at the University of Edinburgh have been researching a possible link between chemicals in the environment and fertility.

  'There is plenty of evidence that if we expose rodents to very high levels of oestrogens, it causes very damaging reproductive effects,' says Professor Sharpe. 'But that is due to the fact that you are suppressing the action of androgens – the male sex hormone. [If you correct that reduction – in other words, you replace the male androgens – it actually doesn't matter how much oestrogen you expose the animals to, they are fine.]'

  Once researchers realised that androgens were the all-important factor, they focused on what sort of environmental chemicals could suppress androgen production by the foetal testis. Top of the list were phthalates. Pronounced 'f-THAL-lates', these chemicals make plastics more flexible and durable, and are hard to avoid as they are used in so many everyday items – from cosmetics to cleaning products, food packaging to fragrance, shower curtains to car dashboards. In fact, phthalates are so ubiquitous that they can be detected in the urine of about 95 per cent of us, and some have suggested a link to all sorts of health conditions, including infertility.

But while subsequent research has shown that phthalates cause reproductive disorders in some animals, such as rats, it suggests that they don't have an effect in humans.

'Our research, and that of others, showed that phthalates had no effect on androgen production by the foetal human testis. And the levels humans are exposed to are at least 25,000 times lower than the doses needed to induce reproductive disorders in rats.'

However, other plastics may be having an effect on male fertility. BPA (Bisphenol-A) is a plastic embedded in all sorts of everyday items, such as water bottles, to make them shatterproof. But it is also known as the 'gender bending' chemical because it has been linked to low fertility. Back in 2010, scientists at research centre Kaiser Permanente in California found that factory workers with higher levels of BPA in their urine were up to four times more likely to have poor semen quality. And a study published in 2018 showed that more than 80 per cent of teenagers from various schools across Devon had traces of BPA in their bodies – despite them trying to avoid it by using glass and steel food and drink packaging.

Another substance to watch out for is glycol ether, which used to exist in paints, glues and printing inks. Since being removed from many products, the risk has reduced, but studies by Professor Pacey and his team at Sheffield University showed that it has an effect on male fertility: 'The risk of men having low motile sperm counts is increased when they are exposed to glycol ether. This should by now have been removed from the supply chain. But just in case it hasn't, then men in occupations risking exposure should be aware of that and use the protective equipment provided, open a window, make sure they get fresh air, that kind of thing.'

- **Air pollution:** Research has shown that air pollution can affect male fertility. One study in Taiwan on 6475 men found that polluting particles affected sperm shape and size. And, in the US, two separate studies also revealed the effect of air pollution – one study showed that it can affect how sperm move, while another showed higher sperm DNA fragmentation in steel plant workers than those not working in the industry. Experts think that pollutants may cause inflammation or that tiny bits of heavy metals may interfere with hormones and mess with DNA.

The main problem is that environmental factors such as plastics, chemicals and pollutants can be tricky to control, particularly if you live in a city or work in a certain industry. Professor Pacey suggests: 'Try to limit your exposure to chemicals and compounds that you are able to control – cosmetic products, plasticisers in shrink-wrapped foods. Just be aware.'

With all of these lifestyle factors, it's worth bearing in mind that as fresh sperm is produced once every 12 weeks, whatever changes you make will take 12 weeks to show any benefit. So, even if you haven't touched a drop of alcohol for months, but then have a very boozy weekend (say, consuming 30–40 units), this binge drinking will affect sperm quality.

## Delayed impact

The problem with your sperm may not be caused by what you're exposed to now, but what you were exposed to when you were in your mother's womb.

Paracetamol is one such concern. Currently, the NHS says it is fine to take paracetamol as a painkiller during pregnancy. But research on the drug by Professor Richard Sharpe and colleagues at the University of Edinburgh has raised concerns.

'Our research showed that paracetamol will suppress testosterone production by the foetal human testis at doses equivalent to those that a pregnant woman would take,' says Sharpe. 'What we don't have an answer to is: how long would the mother need to take paracetamol for, and at what sort of doses, for it to translate into a real reproductive disorder in the developing male.'

The reason scientists don't have an answer is that it is hard to study. Most women will take paracetamol in pregnancy for a day here or there. Large studies would need to be carried out, where paracetamol use is recorded at various stages in pregnancy, and then their children's fertility analysed many years later to see if there is any change related to whether or not their mother used paracetamol when pregnant.

More recently, Professor Sharpe's team has been looking at the effect of paracetamol on both male and female germ cells – the cells that go on to become either sperm or eggs. This research found that paracetamol and ibuprofen reduce the number of germ cells in both male and female rats (and similar findings have been reported in mice). Sharpe and colleagues have also gone on to show that exposure of human foetal ovaries and testes to paracetamol or ibuprofen (at levels equivalent to those that we take) reduces germ cell numbers similar to that found in rats. However, these studies were performed *in vitro* (outside of the body), so they can't be certain about what effects might occur in pregnancy and how much painkiller exposure would be needed to cause any effect.

'Males have the capacity to compensate, as germ cell multiplication is going on all the time throughout life to make sperm,' says Professor Sharpe. 'But when a baby girl is born, she has all the eggs in her ovaries that she will ever have. We know that that is determined fairly early in pregnancy. If you interfere with that at the wrong stage, there is no possibility to correct it. But we have no idea how long you would need to have exposure for, and exactly when during pregnancy, for this to translate into the number of eggs a girl is born with being reduced, which will then determine her reproductive lifespan.'

The hope is that one day a study will be able to determine exactly how paracetamol affects germ cells, so that scientists can then create a painkiller that doesn't use that particular mechanism.

In the meantime, it is important to reiterate that the NHS currently says it is safe to take paracetamol during pregnancy. But mums-to-be need to follow the guidelines, which say that paracetamol should be taken at the minimal dose for the minimum period of time to alleviate symptoms.

## How are you coping?

If you've been trying to conceive for more than a year, the first step is to go and chat to your GP. Officially, your GP won't be able to refer you to a fertility clinic until you've been trying for two years. But it's worth getting some advice and getting the wheels in motion, so that you're ready to be referred. And a reminder that if you are 36 or over (woman) or 40 or over (man) then your GP should refer you sooner.

## Finding out what's wrong

One of the toughest things to deal with in life is not knowing why you're ill or suffering from certain symptoms. This is certainly true with unexplained infertility. Hopefully, by working closely with a consultant at a fertility clinic you'll eventually find an answer. Even if it's bad news, it can be helpful to find out *why* you've been struggling to conceive.

The good news is that for many anatomical issues, there are treatments that can sort out the problem. As Dr Valentine Akande, Medical Director for the Bristol Centre for Reproductive Medicine, says, conditions such as endometriosis, PCOS or hypogonadism don't necessarily mean that you'll never be able to conceive. Most conditions are treatable.

# Dealing with Stress

Experts all say to try to live your regular life as much as possible. Changing your daily routine while going through treatment can increase stress levels and, hence, cause you to slip into bad habits that may affect your fertility. So, as much as possible, remove any stressors from your life and rely on healthy coping mechanisms.

## Professor Jacky Boivin, an expert in developmental psychology at the University of Cardiff, says...

'Take an inventory of your coping strategies. Sometimes, when we encounter new stressors, we forget about all the coping strategies that we used in the past for other challenging times. Maybe you rely on social support. Maybe you solve problems. Maybe you fantasise about an event or thing.'

Boivin recommends checking the impact of fertility problems on your quality of life by completing the online survey FertiQoL (http://sites.cardiff.ac.uk/fertiqol/complete-fertiqol-online/ ), which asks questions such as:

- Do you feel drained or worn out because of fertility problems?
- Do your fertility problems interfere with your day-to-day work or obligations?
- Are you satisfied with your sexual relationship even though you have fertility problems?
- Do your fertility problems cause feelings of jealousy and resentment?
- Do you feel social pressure on you to have (or have more) children?
- Do you feel uncomfortable attending social situations because of your fertility problems?

If you're scoring highly in all these areas, it might be worth chatting to a counsellor (*see* page 103).

'When I first found out we'd need IVF, I was pretty surprised, although I generally felt pretty down about trying to conceive for months beforehand, so it wasn't a significant change to the strain I already felt.' **ANON**

## Cutting back on guilty pleasures

When you're trying to conceive, giving up some of life's little pleasures can be tough. Your usual post-work wind-down routine might have been to have a glass of wine or enjoy a cigarette. As we've seen, these can significantly affect your fertility. So try to find other small things that are healthier yet just as indulgent – maybe a relaxing (not too hot) bath or catching up on the latest series that you love.

If you're struggling to adopt a healthier lifestyle, talk to your partner about how you can both make small changes. Research shows that if one partner changes their lifestyle for more healthy behaviours, such as quitting smoking or eating better, the other is twice as likely to do the same.

## Keep communicating

The key is to stay positive (easier said than done) and keep communicating with your consultant and, crucially, your partner if you have one. You might also find it useful to join online chat forums where others are going through the same challenges and might be able to offer some useful advice, or simply understand how you're feeling.

'I didn't really talk to my friends as I felt like I had nothing to say to them. No one really knows how you feel, so I felt there's not much point.' **NICKY**

▶

'Once I congratulated a friend on his wife falling pregnant. Knowing full well we had male factor infertility, he just shrugged his shoulders and said, "After eight months of trying, I'm just relieved to know I'm fully functional." That decimated my confidence at the time.' **RICHARD**

'There's a huge online community of people trying to conceive and going through IVF. I started my own Instagram IVF account, as I wanted to speak to people. From that I connected with women locally, and we've had several meet-ups, as I wanted to see people face to face. It was nice to speak to others going through the same thing and feel normal.' **ALANA**

## CHAPTER 2

# How IVF works

A step-by-step guide on what to expect from standard IVF and other fertility treatments

Standard IVF usually involves the woman having to take a cocktail of drugs for a number of weeks to control her natural menstrual cycle and boost egg production. The eggs are then extracted from the ovaries, fertilised with the partner's (or donor's) sperm in a glass Petri dish, and then the embryo is reinserted into the womb (uterus).

A typical IVF treatment cycle takes around six to eight weeks, from when you first start taking drugs to the pregnancy test, but this time frame depends on how you respond to the drugs.

'I was most surprised by how common it is for people to require IVF. That was reassuring in some way. I was also surprised by the amount of successful steps that are needed for the process to work and how it could easily have failed at any one of those steps.' VENKI

'There are so many different types of IVF, different drugs, cycles, levels of stimulation, that it was difficult to decipher what would be best for us. At the start of each cycle of IVF, we were left to nurses who were extremely busy, and things often felt rushed. In hindsight, they probably gave us the right answers ▶

and information, but at the time it felt like they could have been clearer, especially as we were very concerned about getting everything right. Although all the doctors and nurses were lovely, it often felt a little bit like a conveyor belt.' **ED**

The treatment is fine-tuned to each patient, but here's a general outline of the steps you're likely to go through once you've chosen a clinic (*see* chapter 3).

## Step 1: Tests

First up, you (and your partner if you have one) will need to have various tests, all of which should give an idea of why you may be struggling to conceive. Your local GP surgery should be able to do some of these, otherwise you'll have to go to a clinic.

The tests for the woman may include a cervical smear test, a urine test or swab for the sexually transmitted infection chlamydia (*see* page 16), and blood tests – one around seven days before your period to measure your progesterone level and check you are ovulating normally, and the second during your period to measure your levels of oestradiol, follicle-stimulating hormone (FSH) and luteinising hormone (LH). But, at any time, the woman can do a blood test for anti-Müllerian hormone (AMH) to find out about their ovarian reserve (the ability of the ovaries to produce eggs), which is actually a more reliable test than checking FSH and LH.

'Once when the hospital had messed up my appointment time by two hours, I had a meltdown in the waiting room. I lost the plot, bursting into tears, and was quickly bundled into a spare office for tea and biscuits!' **SOPHIE**

Men will probably need to have blood tests, and to produce both a urine sample to test for chlamydia and a sperm sample to see whether the sperm is up to scratch. Producing a sperm sample can be quite a challenging moment for a man and may lead to 'performance anxiety' or the inability to ejaculate. Bear in mind that everyone probably feels a bit embarrassed having to perform on cue.

You need to collect the sample directly into a specific container. Don't transfer it from another surface, as that could contaminate it. And you will need to try to collect all the ejaculate to give an accurate indication of sperm count.

You can produce the sample at home, but you'll need to make sure that you've collected a container for the sample from the clinic beforehand, and that you can get your sample to them within one hour. The best way to maintain the sample at body temperature during the journey to the clinic is to keep it in a pocket.

Alternatively, you can produce the sample at the clinic. A nurse will show you to a private room (and obviously then leave!), where there will probably be some 'inspirational' magazines. You produce your sample in the container provided, put it in a see-through bag provided, and deposit that in a hatch in the room, from where the embryologist can retrieve it.

Jheni's story...

The first time Max had to give a sperm sample he didn't properly screw the top back on the sample container before putting it in the see-through bag. The clinic called him that afternoon to explain the 'sticky' situation – and asked him to return to have another go. This was just one of a number of slightly amusing incidents on our IVF journey.

'The "inspirational" literature on offer may not be that "inspiring". When I had to produce my sperm sample at the clinic, I remember the magazines not being that pornographic, and there was an amusing poster on the wall, which showed a huge wave crashing against a lighthouse with the word "Inspire". **MAX**

'When we found out we would need IVF I felt relieved that we finally had an answer and glad to know what the problem was.' **Nicky**

There are some cases where the man needs a helping hand. For example, if he's struggling to ejaculate during masturbation, a latex-free condom can be used to collect sperm during sex with his partner. (Ordinary condoms are designed to be toxic to sperm.) If ejaculation is the problem, the sperm can be removed surgically via an operation collecting them at source from the testes. And, in a small number of cases (such as if there is a neurological issue), through electroejaculation – which is exactly what it sounds like. The patient lies on their side and, usually under general anaesthetic, electrostimulation is applied to a rectal probe. Voltage is gradually ramped up until ejaculation occurs.

And, if in the past a man had a vasectomy, yet he now wishes to try for children, sperm can be taken from his testicles through a technique called surgical sperm recovery, which is carried out either under local or general anaesthetic.

'Before our first consultation I knew very little. I didn't know the difference between IVF and ICSI, I didn't know there would be so many tests, medication and appointments.' **MAX**

## Step 2: Consultation

At your first clinic consultation a few weeks later, your consultant will feed back on your test results. They may also do a scan to get a better idea of any issues with your reproductive system, such as how accessible your ovaries are (in some cases they may be stuck behind the uterus), whether there are any cysts on your ovaries, and if the endometrium is healthy and will be able to support a growing embryo.

You're unlikely to know much about the different treatments or what is involved, so here are some questions to bear in mind that you could ask your clinic consultant. You might want to note down their answers as there could be a lot of information to digest:

- Why am I struggling to get pregnant?
- Is it possible to improve my fertility? If so, how?
- What treatment would you recommend for me – and why do you think it's right for me?
- How does the treatment work?
- Is it accepted by professional bodies?
- How many patients have had this treatment in the last few years – and how many have become pregnant?
- Why do you think other treatments wouldn't be suitable for me?
- If the treatment you've recommended doesn't work, what are the other options available to me after that?
- What tests will I need to undergo before treatment?
- What should I do in advance of treatment?
- When should I start treatment – and what is the schedule?
- Which drugs will I need? And how will they affect my body in terms of side effects?
- How will I take the drugs?
- Are there any alternatives to the drugs you've suggested?
- What is the total cost? And can you give me a cost breakdown?
- Are there any offers available? (Such as three cycles for the price of two)
- Which add-ons is it worth me investing in – and why for me?
- Are there any lifestyle changes that will boost my chances of success?
- Where can I find out answers to any future questions I have?
- Are there any support groups or counsellors I can speak to?
- What support is available if the treatment fails?
- What are the important phone numbers I need to know?
- What's the next step?

Once you've had time to process everything, at a second consultation you'll be able to ask further questions, feed back on what treatment you'd like and discuss other details.

Jheni's story…

I remember feeling stunned at our first consultation when Dr Chandra told me I was running out of eggs. Holding back my tears, I felt so emotional that I didn't process much of what he told us. You may well have a similar experience, where you're given some shocking news and struggle to take in anything you're being told. Or you may be relieved to finally be given a reason why you've not been able to conceive after trying for so long.

'Before our first cycle of treatment, I felt a bit fatalistic, as the odds we were given weren't great. I also felt anxious as there wasn't much else I could do to improve our chance of success.' **MAX**

'We knew very little about the whole process before our first consultation. Given we'd been referred across from a gynaecology department, we hadn't thought about it much or done very much of our own research. So for the first cycle, I felt quite underprepared. I wish I'd known a bit more about the process in advance. While the doctor was clearly very knowledgeable, the appointment was relatively short and, in hindsight, seemed better suited to someone who had a better basic level of understanding of the process. I wish I'd done a lot more reading and investigation in advance, to make better use of the first appointment.' **SOPHIE**

'Before our first consultation I knew almost nothing about IVF and certainly nothing about ICSI. During the NHS cycle, nothing was really explained that clearly, but that was different when we had the private cycles.' **NICKY**

'I wasn't prepared for how hard IVF would be, but we were very lucky and got three rounds funded by the NHS, and staff were so kind, thoughtful and supportive each time. When we finally did get pregnant, the whole service was so considerate, even when the baby was born, recognising that it had not been straightforward for us.' **SUSAN**

## Step 3: Consent forms

Once you've decided which treatment to go ahead with, both you and your partner will be given a whole load of separate consent forms to sign. There is a fair amount of paperwork to plough through, so these forms can be taken away and completed at home.

It's important that the clinic knows your exact wishes for every step of the process, but also that you and your partner are on the same page. You may be surprised to find they have different views on certain issues, so it's worth discussing the questions with your partner before completing the consent forms. Also, situations can change (for example, if a partner dies or a couple splits up), so it's important to have all your personal wishes down in writing. These are not set in stone, though – if you want to, you'll be able to change them at a later date.

On the consent forms you'll be asked to confirm you're happy for:

- your eggs, your partner's sperm and your embryos to be used in your IVF treatment, and that they can be frozen
- your clinic to provide your identifying information to the Human Fertilisation and Embryology Authority (HFEA), where it is stored on a secure database

You may also be asked to confirm:

- if it's all right for your clinic to use any leftover eggs, sperm and embryos for training, such as teaching student embryologists how to handle an embryo in a Petri dish

- what you'd like to do with your eggs, partner's sperm or your embryos if you die or you're not able to make decisions if you become ill
- if you're happy for your identifying information to be shared with your GP or another healthcare professional.

'I tried to take one day at a time [when going through IVF] and not think too far in advance. I meditated every day and was mindful of my thoughts. Meditation helped me hugely to stay grounded and mindful throughout the treatment – and we got a positive result.' **CHAMPA**

## Step 4: Menstrual cycle suppression

If you've been prescribed drugs to boost your egg supply, these can trigger luteinising hormone (LH) to be released too early and bring on premature ovulation. So, first, you'll need to take other drugs to suppress your natural menstrual cycle. It's all about timing everything to perfection.

All the drugs are couriered direct to your door a few days in advance of starting them (regardless of whether you're NHS-funded or paying privately). Keeping them at an optimum temperature is crucial, so you'll have to immediately stash some of them away in the fridge. At a previous appointment, a nurse or consultant should have explained how to administer the drugs, but that may have been a while back and you may not remember everything they said, so make sure you read the labels, and give the clinic a call if you have any queries. The delivery also includes a 'sharps box' for safe disposal of the needles that are used for injections.

The process:

You may be asked to take a progesterone drug on what's known as 'day 19' of the menstrual cycle (day 1 being the start of your last period). It induces a withdrawal bleed and so is used to control the timing of the menstrual cycle.

On 'day 21', you'll start taking another drug – what's known as a 'gonadotropin releasing hormone agonist' (GnRH agonist, *see* 'Fertility drugs', page 73), which works by inhibiting the production of sex hormones. This is to make sure you ovulate at the best time later on. It can be either in the form of a daily injection or as a nasal spray five times a day, for roughly two weeks. (Some clinics may ask you to start GnRH agonists straight after your period.)

The drugs that suppress your natural cycle can often cause side effects, such as hot flushes, insomnia and mood swings. Most of these are very similar to classic menopause-type symptoms, as you're basically undergoing 'temporary menopause'.

Jheni's story…

As far as I can tell I didn't suffer from any of these side effects. (Although Max might not agree!) But I think my body was extra-sensitive at the time, as I remember being away on a camping trip and picking up food poisoning from a barbecue we were sharing with friends. No one else got sick, but I spent a lot of the night over the toilet – not the nicest when you're at an eco-campsite with drop toilets!

## Drugs to control your natural menstrual cycle

These first two drugs control your natural menstrual cycle to ensure that later on in the treatment process you ovulate at the optimum time…

**Gonadotropin-releasing hormone (GnRH) agonists** (such as Buserelin or Goserelin), which block the hormones that regulate your natural menstrual cycle. Buserelin is taken either as a daily ▷

injection or a number of times a day by spraying the drug up your nose. Goserelin is taken as a one-off injection. (*See* page 73 for more on gonadotrophin.)

**Gonadotropin-releasing hormone antagonists** (such as Cetrotide, Orgalutran or Fyremadel), which block the hormone that causes the eggs to be released, preventing ovulation until the eggs are ready to be collected. You take it as a daily injection in your stomach or thigh, starting a few days after starting the gonadotropin injections.

**As the drugs above affect your progesterone levels,** progesterone drugs (such as Crinone, Lubion or Cyclogest) may be prescribed to help thicken the endometrium, meaning the embryo stands a better chance of surviving the first few weeks of pregnancy. Crinone is a vaginal gel, Lubion is injected under the skin, and Cyclogest can be inserted into the vagina as a pessary or into the anus as a suppository (both are roughly the size of a small tampon and can cause sickness or make breasts feel tender).

## Step 5: Egg boost

To stimulate the ovaries to produce more eggs, you'll then need to take an egg-boosting drug, which contains the naturally occurring female hormones FSH (follicle-stimulating hormone) and LH (luteinising hormone). A reminder – FSH prompts follicles to mature, while LH stimulates the most developed follicle to release an egg.

Jheni says…

I took Menopur once a day for at least five days. It comes as a separate liquid and powder that needs to be mixed together, and then injected into the stomach.

When you first do this it can seem slightly complicated (*see* 'How to inject the drug Menopur', box below) and you're likely to feel nervous about injecting yourself. That's completely understandable – most of us have never had to stick a needle in ourselves before. You could ask your partner to do the injection.

Just as with the drugs used to suppress your natural menstrual cycle, a nurse or consultant should have previously explained how to administer these egg-boosting drugs. But if you can't remember, read the medication instructions carefully and call the clinic if you have any queries.

## Jheni's story...

I had a friend who'd been through IVF show me step-by-step how to prepare the egg-boosting drug and do the injection. It hurt a bit, but nothing more than the sting you feel when the needle pierces your skin during a blood test, although the sensation of the liquid entering your flesh can feel a bit odd. But I found that once I'd injected myself a few times, it became a part of my daily routine – no more arduous than brushing my teeth. In all honesty, it sounded worse than it was – by the end all I had was a nice ring of small bruises from the injection points across my tummy, as if someone had drawn a dot-to-dot smiley face under my belly button.

## How to inject the drug Menopur

While some drugs come ready prepared, Menopur requires a few steps of preparation...

### 1) **Prepare the liquid**
Hold the bottom of one of the glass capsules containing the liquid. With the other hand, flick the top of the capsule to ensure all the liquid is at the bottom.

▷

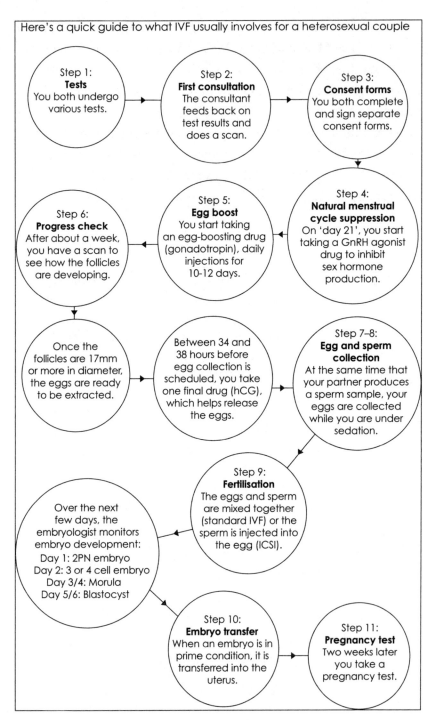

Here's a quick guide to what IVF usually involves for a heterosexual couple

**Step 1:**
**Tests**
You both undergo various tests.

**Step 2:**
**First consultation**
The consultant feeds back on test results and does a scan.

**Step 3:**
**Consent forms**
You both complete and sign separate consent forms.

**Step 4:**
**Natural menstrual cycle suppression**
On 'day 21', you start taking a GnRH agonist drug to inhibit sex hormone production.

**Step 5:**
**Egg boost**
You start taking an egg-boosting drug (gonadotropin), daily injections for 10-12 days.

**Step 6:**
**Progress check**
After about a week, you have a scan to see how the follicles are developing.

Once the follicles are 17mm or more in diameter, the eggs are ready to be extracted.

Between 34 and 38 hours before egg collection is scheduled, you take one final drug (hCG), which helps release the eggs.

**Step 7–8:**
**Egg and sperm collection**
At the same time that your partner produces a sperm sample, your eggs are collected while you are under sedation.

**Step 9:**
**Fertilisation**
The eggs and sperm are mixed together (standard IVF) or the sperm is injected into the egg (ICSI).

Over the next few days, the embryologist monitors embryo development:
Day 1: 2PN embryo
Day 2: 3 or 4 cell embryo
Day 3/4: Morula
Day 5/6: Blastocyst

**Step 10:**
**Embryo transfer**
When an embryo is in prime condition, it is transferred into the uterus.

**Step 11:**
**Pregnancy test**
Two weeks later you take a pregnancy test.

## 2) **Break the capsule**
Place your thumb on the neck of the capsule and press firmly away from you. By being decisive, the capsule neck should break cleanly.

## 3) **Mix the liquid and powder**
Place one of the larger needles on the end of a syringe. Extract the liquid from the open capsule, then pierce the rubber cover on one of the small powder bottles and inject the liquid into it. The powder and liquid will mix – no need to shake.

## 4) **Inject your tummy**
Ensure you swap to a smaller needle. Extract the liquid-and-powder mixture from the bottle. Pinch the skin somewhere around your tummy button and slowly inject the mixture into your skin. Dispose carefully of all needles, capsules and bottles.

In over 90 per cent of treatment cycles, the drug stimulates 6 to 15 follicles to become viable for egg collection. But in some cases, it can overstimulate the ovaries, with potentially dangerous repercussions.

## What is OHSS?

Ovarian hyperstimulation syndrome (OHSS) is when too many follicles or eggs develop in the ovaries, so they swell and become painful. The swelling is due to fluid leaking through the blood vessel walls, which become more permeable from the hormone medication. This can be caused by egg-boosting drugs.

Patients who suffer from OHSS have a higher risk of developing deep vein thrombosis (DVT), so often need to take heparin in advance.

Mild OHSS is fairly common and occurs in about 33 per cent of patients going through fertility treatment. Any problems usually settle down within a few days. For moderate OHSS, patients can take anti-nausea medication and painkillers, and are advised to balance their fluid intake (not drink too much or too little). In rare cases, patients will need to have excess abdominal fluid drained. Just over 1 per cent of women going through IVF will suffer from moderate or severe OHSS.

Severe OHSS can cause you to throw up, and suffer from tummy pain and shortness of breath, and also gain weight rapidly. In severe cases, patients can be prescribed drugs to suppress ovarian activity, or to reduce levels of the hormone prolactin, which can mess with the production of FSH (the key hormone needed to make follicles to mature). Worst-case scenario: a patient might have to be hospitalised in order to be monitored and placed on a drip.

In the past, if a patient had to go to hospital because of OHSS, the clinic had to report it to the HFEA. But the HFEA now requires clinics to alert them to severe cases of OHSS, regardless of whether the patient is hospitalised. This was off the back of a concern that severe cases were being under-reported. Indeed, 60 cases were reported to the HFEA in 2015 and 38 in 2016, compared to the 865 that were actually admitted to hospital for OHSS in England in those years. The Office for National Statistics recorded two deaths from OHSS in England and Wales between 2001 and 2016.

Depending on the severity of OHSS, the consultant may decide to abandon a cycle of treatment prior to egg collection, or may advise to freeze all embryos and defer embryo transfer.

If you ever have any concerns, talk to your consultant or one of the clinic nurses immediately.

At some points in the treatment process there can be a lot of drugs to take in one day. You might find it useful to set alarms to remind you. Ensuring you take the drugs at the right time is one of the things that can be most challenging, as you're still trying to carry on with the usual busy-ness of life – whether that is at work, out at dinner or while on holiday.

## Jheni's story…

I remember sunbathing on a gorgeous Sardinian beach, the sea gently lapping at the shore. An alarm suddenly pierced through this tranquil scene. Myself and fellow sunbathers craned their necks to see who was responsible for the rude interruption. I quickly realised it was the alarm I'd set on my phone to remind me to take the third nasal spray of the day. Fishing the bottle out of a cup filled with sea water (to stop it getting too hot in the baking sun), I proceeded to snort the drugs while watched by irate yet intrigued onlookers. Experiences like these were all just par for the course when going through IVF.

'I was really surprised at all the different types of medication my wife needed to take, and how strict the timing was.' **MAX**

## Egg-boosting drugs

These drugs may increase the number of eggs available for release or ovulation.

**Clomiphene citrate** (such as Clomid or Letrozole) can be used to improve or regulate ovulation by increasing the secretion of follicle-stimulating hormone (FSH), which stimulates follicle development. Starting on the second day of your menstrual cycle, you take tablets for five days. The downside is that the risk of multiple pregnancy is high – between 2 and 13 per cent (*see* page 115 for why many clinics try to avoid multiple pregnancies).

**Gonadotropins** (such as Menopur) contain FSH and luteinising hormone (LH), which help to stimulate the ovaries to produce more eggs, or can help women with PCOS ovulate. They are taken as a daily injection. (If your partner suffers from low levels of gonadotropin hormones – which stimulate sperm production – gonadotropins can be taken to produce more sperm.)

## Step 6: Progress check

After about a week of injecting gonadotropins, you normally have a scan to see how the follicles are developing. As follicles grow, they produce the hormone oestrogen, and sometimes the clinic will also do a blood test to check your oestrogen levels. The aim is to get follicles that are 17mm or more in diameter. Once they've hit this optimum size, they're ready for the eggs to be extracted from them. Between 34 and 38 hours before egg collection, you'll take one final hormone injection of human chorionic gonadotropin (hCG), which helps the eggs to be released.

**This is the injection that you really don't want to mess up.** Depending on the appointment time that you're booked in for to have your eggs collected, you'll be given a very specific time to inject the hCG drug the day before. Don't worry if you're 15 minutes early or late with this final injection. But if it's any more or less, then give the clinic a ring immediately and they'll be able to shift the schedule around to work for you.

Making sure you hit the right time to inject the human chorionic gonadotropin drug can be nerve-wracking.

Jheni's story…

First time we went through IVF, I was at a friend's wedding in Sheffield. At 9:15 p.m. exactly, while everyone else was Gangnam style-ing, I was outside in the car injecting myself with the hCG drug Ovitrelle. Then it was back to the party – no drinking, of course. It all went smoothly, but there was a point where I was thinking I shouldn't be here, too much is at stake, what happens if it all goes wrong. Maybe better to be in the comfort of your own home where you feel more in control of the situation.

'After all the time, energy and cost, I was nervous that making a mistake with one of the injections might reduce our chances.' SOPHIE

## Step 7: Semen collection

So much of the IVF process is focused on the woman – priming your body and checking you're doing all right emotionally. It can be easy to forget just how challenging it must be for the man. Sure, it's the 21st century. But some men might understandably feel emasculated by having to go through fertility treatment. And that's just the psychological challenge. Most (honest) men will tell you that having to perform on cue isn't easy. I say hats off to every guy who has to go into a small room in a clinic and masturbate into a container – all in the short window of opportunity when their partner's eggs have just been extracted and are awaiting the crucial final ingredient.

### Jheni's story...

By the end of the IVF process, Max was pretty relaxed about having to produce semen samples. But there were a couple of hiccups along the way which we just had to laugh about. Probably the most memorable time was on the day of egg collection – the crucial moment where Max had a window of about an hour or so to produce the sperm sample. As we walked into the clinic, I will never forget the face of the nurse who greeted us. Taking one look at right-handed Max, his right arm in a sling from a dislocated collarbone due to a violent karate take-down, she simply said: 'Oh God'!

What else can you really do in that situation but see the funny side, given how high the stakes are – following such a strict regime of medication and knowing that if this cycle didn't work, we'd need to pay thousands next time. The karate take-down could have wrecked it all.

So, we all had a bit of a chuckle – and the nurse subtly whispered that I could always go into the room with him and help out if needed. But there was no need – Max is a talented man and managed to do what he needed to.

'The sign in the sample room said: "Ask for a male nurse if you have any problems producing a sample"!' **ED**

## What to take to the clinic for the egg collection procedure

- Your IVF notes
- A book or something to do – you may have to wait a while if the previous procedure runs over
- A snack
- Water bottle
- Slippers
- Dressing gown – a thin cotton back-fastening gown is provided, but it's nice to have something warm to go over it while you wait
- Comfortable clothes to wear after the procedure as your tummy may be slightly sore afterwards

NB: Do not wear any perfume or body lotion– apparently embryos don't like strong smells.

## Dr Valentine says…

'Perfume is a VOC [volatile organic compound]. It's noxious. It's not that if you wear perfume, you can't get pregnant. It's about marginal gains. It's about not reducing your chance. The embryologists aren't allowed to wear perfume in the clinic.'

## Step 8: Egg collection

Egg collection happens at a very specific time because it's so crucial to get the eggs out when they're in prime condition. The eggs are collected by a needle that is passed through the vagina and into each ovary, guided by ultrasound. In most cases, each follicle is drained and the eggs sucked out. For women like myself who have very few follicles, each one is drained and then flushed out with a fluid. The embryologist then checks under a microscope to see whether an egg has been found. If not, the follicle continues to be flushed and drained, flushed and drained. After four or five attempts, if there's nothing then they accept it's empty and move on.

## Dr Chandra says...

'In some patients, the egg collection process can be technically difficult. For example, if the ovaries are stuck behind the uterus. Or, if somebody has had an infection or appendicitis, and things are stuck inside, you then have to manipulate and press on the abdomen to bring the ovary down. Or if the ovary is behind the uterus, you've got to press, poke and prod a bit. So that can be quite difficult.'

The actual egg extraction should take only about 30 minutes. But, as you have to go under sedation, you will be in the clinic for a couple of hours afterwards while the nurses monitor your recovery. You won't be able to drive yourself home afterwards, so someone will need to come and collect you.

## Jheni's story...

Before undergoing egg collection for the first cycle of IVF, I remember being most nervous about having a general anaesthetic. For some reason I was fixated on this, instead of worrying about whether we were going to get lucky and retrieve some eggs, whether any would fertilise, whether one would be viable and eventually lead to a pregnancy... No, it was all about whether I was going to wake up OK. I'd never been under general before, and for some reason I didn't like the idea of not being in control. But maybe I was actually subconsciously trying to distract myself from the fact that we'd put so much into this already. ▶

In times of stress, we so often find humour in small things. Driving into the packed car park, I remember Max joking about it being OK to pull up in the 20-minute drop-off parking zone, as that's what we were essentially doing that day – dropping off some eggs and sperm. Then it was an 'au revoir' kiss and see you on the other side. Max was led off to the small sample-depositing room, and I was led into a room where a number of other patients were each waiting in separate bays. Dressed in an operation gown, I was eventually led through to the treatment room. A raised bed sat in the centre, surrounded by various trolleys of equipment. After lying down on the bed, the team checked my blood pressure and I was hooked up to a heart rate monitor. I remember spotting a large hatch on the far wall – I presumed for passing the eggs to the embryology team. The anaesthetist was chatting to me – the usual questions – name, date of birth...

That's the one thing you get asked a lot – at every stage of the process, whenever you meet a new team member, the first question they ask is your name and D.O.B. This is to be absolutely sure that the right egg is paired with the right sperm. The clinic where we went through IVF treatment now has some software that cross-checks the couples' details.

Waking from my deep slumber, I remember one of the first people to come to my bedside was our consultant, Dr Chandra. In his wonderful mild manner, he asked how many eggs I would hope he had collected. I remember reaching for his hand and saying, 'I'd just be delighted with one!' Naively, I thought one egg would do the trick. Fortunately, Dr Chandra had managed to get out four.

Now, in reality, one egg is pretty unlikely to lead to a baby. Yes – it does only take one egg and one sperm to make a baby. But that one egg has to fertilise, then develop well over the next few days into a quality embryo, then implant successfully and then develop into a baby – avoiding miscarriage...

While the average number of follicles produced in an IVF cycle is usually around 10 to 12, the key thing is the quality of each egg. So, even if you've only got one good-quality embryo, there is always a chance it will result in a successful pregnancy.

> 'I felt the most pressure on the day of egg collection as, first I had to be supportive to my wife, and then I had a 20–30 minute window to provide my sample.' MAX

## Step 9: Fertilisation

In standard IVF, an embryologist immediately mixes the collected eggs with the male sperm in a Petri dish – not a test tube. (The term 'test tube baby' that was used in the early days wasn't technically correct.) In natural conception, only about two dozen sperm make it to the egg. But in IVF, around 100,000 sperm are placed with the egg in the Petri dish.

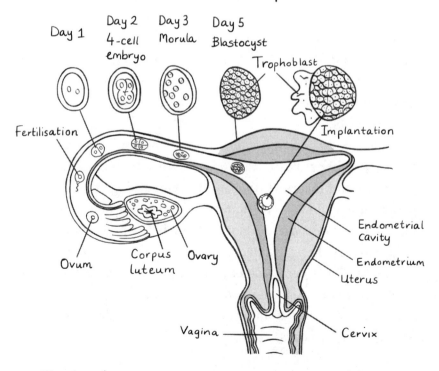

Fertilisation and Implantation

Timeline showing the development of an embryo to a blastocyst

Over the next few days, the embryologists keep a close eye on proceedings. Just as with egg extraction, the work is incredibly skilled – they use pipettes that are just 1mm in diameter to pick up and manoeuvre the developing embryos.

Day 1 after fertilisation, each healthy embryo will still be a single cell, known as two-pronuclear (2PN) embryos. Around 80–90 per cent of mature eggs will develop into 2PN embryos. By day 2, embryos will have three or four cells. By day 3, an ideal embryo will have six, seven or eight cells. Any less or more and it's known as a substandard embryo. Too many cells means that the embryo is growing too fast and using up energy stores, while too few cells and it's unlikely to divide enough for implantation.

By day 3, embryologists can grade embryos on their quality. Top-quality eggs are either A-grade or B-grade. Poor-quality eggs are C-grade, and show a lot of what's known as 'fragmentation', whereby too many fragments mean the cells are not dividing correctly.

The aim is for an embryo to develop to day 5 or 6, when it becomes what's known as a blastocyst. This is around a tenth of a millimetre in diameter and made up of several hundred cells, with a texture that looks a bit like a quilt and a clear mass of cells inside, known as the 'inner cell mass'.

Around 16–20 hours after fertilisation, the clinic will call you to confirm whether any eggs have been fertilised. These calls happen daily at around the same time and the embryologist reports back on how the embryos are doing. Research has shown that the longer the embryos can develop in the lab, the greater the chance at a pregnancy. For a woman aged 35, the chances of pregnancy increase by 10 per cent each day the eggs remain in the incubator post-fertilisation. A blastocyst will be about twice as likely to result in a pregnancy as a morula (an embryo made up of 16 cells after three to four days).

## Jheni's story…

On our first cycle of IVF, of the four eggs that, Dr Chandra managed to retrieve, all had fertilised – but only three normally and one 'atypically' (meaning it wasn't viable) – and only one made it to blastocyst stage.

I remember the days immediately after egg extraction and before transfer being tough. It's hard not to get excited every day when the embryologist calls for an update on the embryos, but also nervous in case it's not good news and there are no viable embryos to transfer. On day 5 the embryologist called to tell me the good news that there was one high-quality grade-A embryo. The not-such-good news was that neither of the other two embryos had continued developing overnight and so weren't high enough quality to warrant freezing (see page 166 for more on freezing your eggs or embryos) – for a potential second go if this cycle failed.

I remember I was standing in a stationery cupboard – the only quick access private place near enough to my desk in an office I was working in at the time. The printer humming in the background, surrounded by shelves of paper, pens, staplers, folders, scissors (and the typical paraphernalia that you never quite know why the receptionist has ordered), I remember hearing this news and feeling devastated that I only had one embryo. It had all seemed to be going so well just yesterday with three good ones remaining.

The embryologist obviously heard the disappointment in my voice and quickly tried to reassure me, telling me to focus on the fact that we had one really high-quality embryo to work with. It made me realise what a tough job staff at clinics have – to be factually correct, not raise hopes, and yet be caring and sensitive to every couple. The embryologist did her job so well that I ended the call buoyed up again and ready for embryo transfer the next morning.

## Paul Wilson, BCRM Head of Embryology and Andrology, says...

'In the lab, what we're trying to do is to mimic the environment the embryo would encounter in the body and ensure we do not introduce any form of contamination. For example, with eggs and embryos, we know if we deviate from body temperature for anything more than a very short period of time, and by anything more than a degree or so, we can affect the future viability of the embryo, because the delicate structures within the cells may be affected. So we work on heated surfaces, and the lab air background air quality is highly purified to remove airborne contaminants.

'Immediately after egg extraction, we empty the contents of the test tube into a Petri dish, quickly identify the presence of the egg using the microscope and then wash the egg to remove any blood that may be present as this can inhibit fertilisation.

'The sperm sample comes into the other side of the lab, or if it has been previously frozen, we thaw it. We prepare the sperm in a way that allows us to end up with a concentrated pellet of the best-quality sperm, which we then use to attempt fertilisation. As we're not interested in any of the other cells and fluids of the ejaculate, or any dead sperm, these are removed during processing, usually using a technique called density gradient separation; this is rather like a liquid sieve, where the sperm is put on top of different concentrations of solutions containing very small particles and then centrifuged at about 400 times the force of gravity, which creates the concentrated pellet. The preparation process can be viewed as mimicking the action of the cervix, because dead sperm in the ejaculate will never pass through the cervical mucus, which acts like a filter. Sperm are incredibly hardy and can withstand some rather amazing conditions without their fertilisation potential being impacted.

'Then we put the sperm and the eggs together, either via IVF or ICSI. Next morning, about 16 to 18 hours later, we hope to see the signs of fertilisation. What we're looking for is the nucleus of the egg and the nucleus of the sperm, known as 'pronuclei'; they resemble two small balls within the centre of the embryo. If we see three pronuclei, this is an abnormal fertilisation, perhaps caused by two sperm fertilising the egg at the same time, resulting in an incorrect number of additional chromosomes. We may also see no change – the egg has failed to fertilise, or we may see atypical fertilisation, where we see only parts of the signs of fertilisation, for example a single pronucleus.

'The signs of fertilisation are short-lived, so it is important we carry out these observations at the right time. As the signs are transient, if we were to carry out assessments outside of the correct windows, this could have serious repercussions for the treatment outcome; an abnormally fertilised embryo can potentially develop like a typically fertilised embryo, all the way to the blastocyst stage, and be selected for transfer or storage.

'Once we've created the embryos, our focus changes to selection; we aim to identify which is/are the best embryo(s) from the group of available embryos. Traditionally, one would take an embryo dish out of the incubator once or twice a day to make assessments; it's like a snapshot in time. But you're making those assessments based on what you see at that particular moment, and you're exposing the embryos to air, light and temperature changes. Time-lapse incubation allows us to leave the embryo dish in the machine, take a picture of the embryo using a high-powered microscope every 10 to 15 minutes, 24 hours a day. We can then string these images together to create a video, which shows us things that may take place in the dead of night and may help us to identify the best embryos more easily. What we can't do, of course, is make non-viable embryos viable, but we can hope to reduce the time and number of treatments required to achieve a pregnancy.'

## TESTING FOR GENETIC DISEASES

If you or a family member have a serious genetic condition, you might want to find out whether your embryos also have that condition to avoid your children inheriting it. Pre-implantation genetic diagnosis (PGD), or pre-implantation genetic testing (PGT-M), is a technique used to check an embryo's genes for a particular genetic condition. It involves taking a cell or a few cells from an embryo and screening them for genes linked to the genetic condition. Any embryos without faulty genes can then either be frozen or transferred to the uterus.

The number of patients using PGD is relatively small, but identification of serious inherited conditions has risen in recent years.

Your clinic can offer counselling to help you decide your course of treatment. The Genetic Alliance is also a good resource to help make decisions (*see* page 104).

**Step 10: Embryo transfer**

When the embryologist deems it the optimum moment, the best one or two embryos are chosen for transfer. The actual embryo transfer process only takes about 20 minutes, because all it involves is putting the embryo back in the uterus. If you've been through a cervical screening test, it's no worse than that.

You'll sit on a special reclining seat, legs akimbo, a sheet protecting your modesty. If your partner is present, they sit on a chair nearby (as far away as possible from the business site in Max's case). The consultant or a nurse transfers the embryo to the uterus using a catheter passed through the vagina. The catheter is extracted and analysed under a microscope to double-check that it is empty and that the embryo has remained in the uterus.

To plump up the endometrium for implantation, you'll probably be given extra progesterone in the form of either a gel, an injection, a pessary or a suppository to take every 12 hours, starting a few days in advance of embryo transfer. NICE guidelines say there's no point in doing an embryo transfer if the endometrium is less than 5mm thick as it is unlikely to result in a pregnancy.

The number of embryos transferred usually depends on your age. According to NICE, under the age of 37 a single embryo should be transferred in the first cycle, and the same for the second cycle unless there are no top-quality embryos, when two could be considered, and in the third cycle a maximum of two should be transferred. The same goes for women aged between 37 and 39 years, except a double embryo transfer could be considered for the first cycle if there are no top-quality embryos. A double embryo transfer should be considered for women over 40 from the first cycle.

Dr Chandra says…

'The age of the female partner is the most important criterion, because that determines success rates. Between age 41 and 42, and 42 and 43, there is an enormous difference. In a patient who is 30, the risk of a miscarriage is about 15 per cent because of chromosomal abnormalities. But, at age of 45, the chance of a natural conception is less than 5 per cent. But, of those less than 5 per cent, the risk of a miscarriage is about 85 per cent. So if her chance of conception is only 1–2 per cent and the risk of miscarriage at age 45 is 85 per cent, then those that get pregnant naturally and go to term and have a baby are few in number.'

Dr Chandra says…

'Embryo transfer is one of the most crucial procedures in fertility treatment. It's important to do it gently and precisely under ultrasound guidance. The most common things that patients ask straight after are: When I stand up, will the embryo fall out? No. If I go to the toilet, will the embryo fall out? No. Do I need to lie down? No. But if it makes you happy, you should.'

'I hadn't realised how many hurdles there were to go through. It's not straightforward. There are lots of steps to even get to the celebration of making an embryo.' ALANA

Many people might think that the odds of a successful pregnancy are higher if two embryos are transferred, rather than just one. But research suggests that transferring one embryo is just as successful as transferring two. Between January and December 2015, for example, the Bristol Centre for Reproductive Medicine (BCRM) had just over a 60 per cent success rate with single blastocyst transfer, and just under 50 per cent success with double blastocyst transfer. And a study of 1500 women who were treated at the Nurture Fertility clinic in Nottingham found that transferring two embryos – one of good quality and one poor – cut the chances of getting pregnant by 27 per cent, the reason being that poor-quality embryos are normally rejected by the endometrium. So, if a poor-quality embryo is put back in with a good one, it's more likely to compromise the chance of the good one implanting.

In any case, the HFEA discourages multiple pregnancies (twins, triplets or more) as they are the single greatest health risk to both mothers and babies (*see* page 115). Due to the known health risks to both mother and baby, reducing multiple birth rates has been a key goal of the HFEA for the last decade. It seems to be working, as the latest HFEA stats show that multiple births have dropped from around a quarter IVF births in 2008 to 8 per cent in 2018.

Pretty much straight after embryo transfer, you'll be able to leave the clinic. While you might want to take just take a few minutes in the waiting room before heading home, NICE guidelines say that resting for more than 20 minutes after embryo transfer doesn't improve your chances. Clinics tend to advise against swimming or having a bath for three days.

## Step 11: Pregnancy test

You'll have to wait two weeks before taking a pregnancy test. This is one of the toughest times in the whole process. Some people take a week off work to chill out, although research suggests it's best to stick to your usual routine as much as possible, while not overdoing it. Do what you think is best for you.

## Jheni's story…

The first time we went through IVF, while I didn't rush around, I made sure that I kept myself fairly busy – distraction being a good tonic. Although, throughout those two weeks I was constantly checking every few hours to see if my period had started. Each day without bleeding felt like a huge achievement.

After a long two-week wait, I remember taking the pregnancy test in the bathroom at home. Removing the stick from the packaging, I placed the end in a cup full of urine, and waited. After about 5 minutes, heart thudding in my chest, I looked at the test strip on the stick.

The line was obvious. After years of trying, having always seen a negative result, I couldn't quite believe it. So I took another test.

I was all too aware that this positive result was very early days, and pregnancy can be littered with possible pitfalls. I remember a friend who had been through IVF describing the whole process like a hurdle race. After each step, another barrier had been hurdled, and then another, and then another – until, finally, the finish line looms into sight.

A few weeks after your home pregnancy test, the clinic will call you in to do a scan. It's still early days, but you will be able to see a blob of a foetus on the ultrasound monitor and often hear a heartbeat. Usually the clinic will then refer you to the NHS maternity services, and from this point on you will be treated just like anyone else who is pregnant. It can be hard making the adjustment from being in a specialist IVF clinic to being just another pregnant woman. But if you have any concerns, you can always contact your GP or midwife. Bear in mind that pregnancy can sometimes not be easy. Morning sickness (which actually lasts all day and night), heartburn and extreme fatigue are just some of the symptoms that can plague the early weeks of pregnancy – or the whole way through. While those who have conceived naturally may have a good moan about these hardships, you may feel you're just so lucky to be pregnant following IVF treatment that you shouldn't complain. Just remember not to be too hard on yourself. Getting pregnant for most people is the start of a new journey. To those of us who have been through IVF, we've already run a marathon to get to this point.

Usually people who get pregnant naturally wait until the 12-week scan to start celebrating and telling friends and family. But at six weeks, I told a few close family and friends straight away as they knew we were going through the process. I remember always adding a caveat on the end of the news. I was worried that something could go wrong. Of course things do regularly go wrong in pregnancy and beyond. But as a friend pointed out to me, even once they're born, you never stop worrying about your child. It almost becomes worse as their personality develops, your lives grow more intertwined and your love deepens.

## A FAILED CYCLE

Regardless of the result of the pregnancy test, the clinic like to know the outcome. If it's positive, it'll be an easy call to make. But if it's negative, you may need a bit of time before you feel ready to make that call. Even if you've experienced bleeding during those two weeks, the clinic will ask you to take a pregnancy test, as you could still be pregnant. They may also want to do a scan to ensure that you haven't got an ectopic pregnancy (where the embryo implants in the fallopian tubes rather than in the womb) as there is a slightly higher risk of this if you have IVF.

You will probably be asked to have a follow-up consultation of some sort, which might be over the phone or face to face. It's worth doing this, as it helps to provide closure to the treatment process. Turn to chapter 6 to find tips for how to cope if IVF hasn't worked, and advice from those who have been through a number of failed cycles.

'I was most surprised by the intensity of the process – having to attend almost daily check-up appointments, structuring our lives around injections, awaiting calls every afternoon to get blood results and confirm whether to adjust the dosage, and all the emotion and stress. I think I underestimated how much energy and positivity would be needed. I was also surprised at the length of recovery time I felt I needed after a failed cycle – it seemed ages before I felt ready to try again.' SOPHIE

'Before starting IVF, I knew that it was expensive and could take many cycles to get a positive result. I wasn't aware there were different forms of treatments available. We decided that we were prepared to go through three treatments and then reassess.' CHAMPA

## OTHER FERTILITY TREATMENTS

You may have heard all sorts of other acronyms being bandied around, from ICSI to IUI. In this section you'll find explanations of some of these other fertility treatments.

### WHAT IS ICSI?

For around half of couples who are struggling to conceive, it's the male sperm that causes the problem. If this is the case, intracytoplasmic sperm injection (ICSI) is a solution. ICSI works exactly the same as IVF, except during fertilisation the sperm is injected directly into the egg, as opposed to them just being put in the same Petri dish. This saves the sperm from having to burrow through the egg's outer layer (zona pellucida). The technique is ideal for 'lazy' sperm that aren't good swimmers, if their numbers are low, any of the male reproductive anatomy is damaged or blocked, meaning the sperm can't get through, or there are high levels of anti-sperm antibodies, which hinder their ability to swim or fertilise.

An analysis of Max's semen showed that he didn't have any of these antibodies, but a few 'suboptimal' results suggested that his sperm were not quite up to scratch in other ways.

Max's sperm were slightly on the lazy side at 22 per cent 'progressive motility'. The percentage of normal sperm was 3 per cent – just below the recommendation. And, as the average sperm concentration can go up to 200 million per millilitre, his sperm had a marginally low sperm count of 70 million/ml. But sperm quality can vary substantially in the space of just a few months (*see* chapter 1 for what can be done to improve it). This is because new sperm are produced continually in the testes, taking about four to six weeks to mature. So we decided to wait before starting treatment, and three months later, Max produced another sample for analysis. The results differed in some ways. This time round, sperm concentration was just 14.3 million per millilitre, percentage of normal forms just 2 per cent and total count 35.75 million. So, Max and I were advised to do ICSI.

While IVF mixes around 100,000 sperm with one egg, the ICSI process needs just a few to select the best from. Under a microscope, a single sperm is picked by the embryologist. Then, using a very fine hollow glass needle, less than the width of a human hair, a sperm is injected into the egg's cytoplasm – the fluid material inside the egg. Ensuring that the nucleus is at the top of the egg, the embryologist inserts the needle from the side, so that it doesn't interfere with any of the genetic material in the nucleus. As the egg membrane is very elastic, the needle compresses the egg as it enters, squashing it into a kidney-bean shape. The egg membrane then immediately closes up the hole pierced by the needle, sealing the sperm inside.

Paul Wilson says…

'With IVF, looking at it very simply, we're just observers who provide the right environment for fertilisation and embryo development to take place. The IVF technique is used where there are no identified concerns regarding the sperm or the eggs' ability to interact with each other and we may be, for example, aiming to overcome a mechanical barrier to conception, such as missing fallopian tubes. With IVF, the sperm and egg still have to work their magic; the sperm still have to swim to the eggs, recognise them, the eggs and sperm have to interact and the sperm has to be capable of penetrating the egg. Usually, the sperm binds to the outside of the egg and only the contents of the sperm head (containing the DNA) goes into the egg, with the tail being left behind.

'The ICSI process is a more invasive technique and is advised where there are concerns that fertilisation may not be successful if standard IVF techniques were used. We insert a needle, containing the whole sperm (including the fluid that the sperm is sitting in) into the egg, in an attempt to fertilise the egg. We need to do this very delicately. As ICSI is more invasive, we aim to use it only where we believe it will confer a benefit. The very latest published evidence from the national registers of several countries suggests that ICSI does not lead to improved outcomes over IVF where there is not a clearly identified sperm issue.'

ICSI was developed at Vrije Universiteit Brussel, and the first baby to be born through ICSI was in 1992. Since then, thousands of children have been conceived this way. The technique has really high success rates – fertilisation occurs in about 96 per cent of cases, giving at least twice the chance of a pregnancy than the average fertile couple can hope for each month. But lots of factors still affect a successful pregnancy, such as the woman's age and whether she has any fertility difficulties herself. Interestingly, use of ICSI dropped between 2014 and 2017 (according to the latest HFEA trends report published in 2019). Published research of short-term studies shows it's a really safe technique, but the long-term effects on children conceived in this way are as yet unknown. And it's currently slightly more expensive than standard IVF – an extra £500 to £1000 on top of the standard IVF costs (*see* page 110 for a run-through of average costs).

## WHAT IS IUI?

During intra-uterine insemination (IUI), sperm are injected into your uterus using a fine plastic straw and left to fertilise your eggs naturally. Before doing so, the sperm are washed to weed out the lower quality ones that would move slowly or not at all, and then the remaining fast-movers are injected into your uterus.

As with any fertility procedure, timing is crucial. If you're not using fertility drugs, blood or urine tests will identify when you're due to ovulate, and then IUI will be performed around 12 to 16 days after the first day of your last period.

If you are using fertility drugs to boost egg production and stimulate ovulation, the date you're due to ovulate will be predicted with ultrasound scans and blood tests to monitor LH levels.

IUI is often used by female same-sex couples, single women, or heterosexual couples where the woman has irregular periods, the couple can't have sex, or the man doesn't produce viable sperm so donor sperm is used instead. IUI is also recommended in specific cases, such as if the woman's cervical mucus contains high levels of antibodies to sperm, or if the man suffers from HIV and so sperm washing reduces the risk of passing the disease on to yourself or your baby.

It's worth bearing in mind that the latest figures from the Human Fertilisation and Embryology Authority show that without fertility drugs, 10.8 per cent of women under 35 get pregnant with their partner's sperm through IUI, whereas 12.9 per cent get pregnant when using fertility drugs.

Once the eggs are ready, if you are using fertility drugs then a human chorionic gonadotropin (hCG) drug will be injected to trigger ovulation, and within 38 hours the eggs will be released into the fallopian tubes. Then the sperm is injected into the uterus, which is no more tricky or painful than a smear test. A speculum is inserted into your vagina to keep the walls apart and the sperm is injected through a thin tube called a catheter. Just as with standard IVF, to plump up the endometrium ready for implantation, you'll probably have been given a gel, injection or a pessary containing progesterone. Side effects of taking the pessaries can make you feel a bit sick or your breasts might become slightly tender – which can be confused with being pregnant.

IUI is only given to women with healthy fallopian tubes. Blockages are spotted either using an X-ray or an ultrasound probe. Alternatively, to check the tubes a 'laparoscopy' is performed, where a thin tube with a light and camera on the end is inserted through a small incision in the abdomen while you're under general anaesthetic.

The benefits of IUI are that it is less invasive than IVF (as your eggs don't have to be extracted), it requires fewer drugs and is much less expensive – one cycle of IUI costs between £350 and £1000. But IUI is about a third as successful as IVF. This is because, for example, with IVF you can select the embryos. And, as always, the chances of success depend on the woman's age, the sperm quality and the reasons for low fertility. For women under 35, about 18 per cent are successful with IUI. Between the ages of 35 and 37, success rates are about 14 per cent, 12 per cent between 38 and 39, 5 per cent between 40 and 42, and 1 per cent if over 42.

Also, the risk of multiple pregnancy through IUI (with fertility drugs) is quite high – about 75 per cent single children, 23 per cent twins and 2–3 per cent triplets. So, if more than three mature follicles develop as a result of the fertility drugs, the advice tends to be to ditch the technique. After a number of attempts (which can be as many as eight or nine cycles), couples are normally advised to try IVF or ICSI.

'I was most surprised by how long it all takes and how expensive it is. Before starting IVF, I was nervous about it not working and what my wife would have to go through treatment-wise. But I was mostly nervous that it would get to the point of her wanting to try a sperm donor, which is not something I wanted to do.' NICKY

## HOW NATURAL CYCLE IVF WORKS

Natural cycle IVF is where no drugs are used at any point in the process. Egg collection happens just like with standard IVF, except only one will be collected as this is the one you release naturally during ovulation.

With the current trend towards a more natural, organic lifestyle, natural cycle IVF might sound appealing, but there are a lot of things to consider.

A benefit of natural cycle IVF is that one cycle is cheaper than standard IVF, as you don't have to buy any fertility drugs. But, if it doesn't work first time, you will have to undergo a second full cycle of IVF, rather than potentially being able to use a frozen embryo from the first cycle, so it might actually work out more expensive in the long run.

Not taking fertility drugs means you won't be at risk of any potential side effects from the drugs.

And, because your ovaries aren't being stimulated, your body won't have to take a break after IVF, so you can try again sooner if you want to.

But the flip side is that the timing of egg collection is unpredictable. And the HFEA says that birth rates are currently lower than for standard IVF – the latest stats show it's around 7.5 per cent lower for all ages. Also, at the moment, natural cycle IVF is not recommended by NICE.

## HOW NATURAL CYCLE MODIFIED IVF WORKS

This is a form of natural cycle IVF, which also involves egg collection during the natural menstrual cycle, but some drugs are taken around day 5 or 6 to stop spontaneous ovulation, and a small dose of stimulation hormone ensures follicles remain healthy and continue to grow. Success rates are slightly higher than with natural cycle IVF.

## HOW MILD STIMULATION IVF / IVF LITE WORKS

Mild IVF is just like a standard antagonist cycle of IVF, which uses a much lower dose of gonadotropins (which help to stimulate the ovaries to produce more eggs). The main aim of taking fewer drugs is to get a milder response from the ovaries, so you don't produce too many eggs, which can cause ovarian hyperstimulation syndrome (OHSS) – *see* page 71.

The HFEA currently doesn't have any stats on success rates of mild stimulation IVF. While the majority of patients won't experience any degree of OHSS, if you already know you're prone to OHSS, then it might be worth considering this treatment. Indeed, a study published in 2014 recommended that for women undergoing IVF where more than 15 eggs are collected and the risk of OHSS is high without improving pregnancy success rates, the clinic should offer a lower level of egg-boosting drugs.

Natural cycle IVF and mild IVF are certainly hot topics in the fertility world and a continuing discussion point between experts. Good clinics will always just want the best for their patients and tailor the amount of drugs accordingly. And different clinics offering the same treatment may simply call it different things, such as 'mild IVF' instead of 'standard antagonist cycle of IVF.'

In my case, there would have been no point in trying natural cycle IVF as I didn't produce many eggs, but the ones I did produce were good quality. So, the second time I went through IVF, we bumped up the dose of the egg-boosting drug and I got more good-quality eggs.

The key thing to bear in mind is that everybody's body is different. To ensure that you feel happy you're being offered the best treatment for you, it's worth doing plenty of research into different clinics and what they offer – *see* chapter 3. You might decide that natural cycle modified IVF or mild IVF is the right route for you if *your* fertility is not a problem but your partner's sperm is the reason you're struggling to conceive, or if you froze your eggs while waiting to meet The One, or you're a single person or a female same-sex couple using donor sperm.

Professor Geeta Nargund, Medical Director, CREATE Fertility, says…

'IVF was first invented to help women who had blocked or damaged tubes to have a baby by bypassing the fallopian tubes. Now, IVF is used to help a wide range of women achieve their dream of having a baby, including those who have no fertility problems themselves, such as single women, female same-sex couples, women who want to freeze their eggs for the future, and also in couples with male factor infertility. This means that more and more fertile and healthy women are undergoing fertility treatments. As a society, we should celebrate the diversity we can create by helping single women and the LGBT community start families through IVF. But it's important that, as we get closer to achieving gender equality in fertility treatments, we reduce the burden of such treatments on women. We need to work towards helping women have a baby with fewer drugs, fewer complications and thus, a lower burden of IVF treatment.

Dr Valentine says…

'The interpretation of mild IVF varies depending on whom you speak to. This can include using lower doses of medication or aiming to achieve a lower number of eggs. But the key with any treatment is to do *appropriate* stimulation, and tailor the dose and type of treatment according to individual circumstances. The chances of normal fertilisation with healthy sperm are around 60–70 per cent. In order to optimise the chances of success, it is useful to have more than one embryo to choose from – more eggs help create more embryos and therefore increase the chances of having a baby. Routinely using mild stimulation during IVF treatment results in fewer eggs, fewer embryos, a reduced chance of having embryos to freeze, and a lower chance of having a baby. Therefore more IVF treatments are required to obtain the same chances of success compared to conventional/appropriate IVF, where embryos have a higher chance of being frozen and stored for later use. The research evidence is very clear in this respect: if you use mild stimulation for every patient you will get poorer cumulative pregnancy rates and lower cumulative chances of having a baby.'

## HOW IN-VITRO MATURATION (IVM) WORKS

This is a fairly new technique where your immature eggs are collected from your ovaries and left to mature in the lab, which means you don't have to take any fertility drugs. The eggs are then fertilised via ICSI.

As the HFEA only have records of 13 cycles of IVM (from 2015 to 2017), they are unable to give reliable success rates, and say more research is needed before they confirm the safety of IVM.

### How are you coping?

Going through IVF can be overwhelming – from your first consultation where there's a lot of information to get your head around, through to the ups and downs you're likely to experience along the way.

You may well have a consultation where you're given some shocking news and so struggle to take in everything you're being told. Or maybe you find out that you're the one in the couple with fertility issues. Or perhaps you're relieved to finally be given a reason why you've not been able to conceive after trying for so long. Whatever ▶

your scenario, it might be worth seeing a therapist/counsellor before you start the actual IVF treatment. Again, most clinics will have someone who they can recommend.

## Seeking support

It can be an enormous shock to discover you have fertility issues.

'If a couple is expecting to be given some simple explanation and a few fertility drugs or something, and then the woman discovers that she has only a few, or no eggs, the shock can be huge,' says Wendy Martin, Fertility Therapist at the Bristol Centre for Reproductive Medicine (BCRM). 'For example, if the woman is 32 and has already been through [premature] menopause [possibly without realising] or has been diagnosed with premature ovarian insufficiency (POI), it's a real shock. Likewise, if a man has sperm, but the quality or quantity is so low they are told they will need assisted conception treatment, such as ICSI, and that they will have only one free go at it on the NHS, the shock is tremendous. It can be really hard for this news to sink in.'

Once over the initial news, some couples seek counselling before going through treatment. But different couples want counselling at different times and for different reasons – some when they find out they have a problem with fertility, or when they are about to start treatment, and others when the treatment doesn't result in a pregnancy.

NICE recommends that counselling should be offered before, during and after IVF treatment regardless of the outcome, and the HFEA recommend that each clinic should have at least one person who is trained in infertility counselling.

Whatever your situation, just make sure that you're kind to yourself and your partner. It could be easy to blame one another if you find out one of you has the fertility issue. And don't beat yourselves up if you get a bit teary during the consultation. The consultants are very used to seeing

▶

emotional patients. It's really normal. And don't worry if you don't take everything in – you can always give the consultant a call later on to ask more questions.

'IVF has definitely affected my mental health – it probably still does. I have coping mechanisms – if I have a bad day, I don't put pressure on myself to go to a social event.' **ALANA**

'At an open day at a fertility centre, nobody wanted to talk about their experiences – despite being men who had exactly or very similar life experiences. [With no one to talk to] I wrote a diary of everything that happened to us, which helped. It's not just to help you keep track of what's going on, but also how you feel. Good things. But also bad stuff. It doesn't matter how grim it is. Don't hold back. If you're feeling really crap about something, then write it down. And if blue language pops into your head, then use it. I found it quite cathartic.' **RICHARD**

## Deciding on treatment

With so many different treatment options available, it can be hard to decide which one is best for you. Obviously, in some cases you won't have much choice - for example, if your partner's sperm is sluggish, your clinic will probably advise you to go for ICSI. Before you decide on a treatment, just make sure you've done your research, so that you can feel confident you're making the right decision for you, your body and your potential family. To help you make those sorts of decisions, it's worth drawing up a list of pros and cons, such as the costs (see page 110 for a summary of costs), how invasive the procedure is, or the likelihood of conceiving.

You may be told you need to consider using a donor egg. If you have to decide whether to use donated eggs or sperm, it is likely to be a big decision. It might be helpful to chat to friends and family or a counsellor before making a decision. Most clinics will have a therapist/counsellor who they can recommend. It's worth bearing in mind that hundreds of very happy families are created every year through egg or sperm donation.

The next big step in the treatment process is taking the drugs, which can have side effects, such as mood swings. Before starting treatment, it might be worth chatting with your partner to explain that you might have a few Jekyll-to-Hyde moments and be a little more emotional than normal – and need even more of their support and love.

Going through IVF is such a big deal emotionally and financially that it can be hard not to just focus on that and cut out lots of things in your life. Yes, you need to ensure you're giving your body the best chance, so you don't want to overdo things. But consultants advise you not to make big changes in your life – and to carry on as much as possible with your usual routine.

## Jheni's story…

Max and I tried hard to carry on with life, and not get too obsessed about going through IVF. We kept doing all the usual things that make us happy – walks in the countryside, seeing family and friends, going out for dinner. Yet it was a balancing act to not over-stress my body. The same weekend that we were at the Sheffield wedding I mentioned earlier another very close friend was getting married in Spain. Months before, I'd booked us on a crack-of-dawn flight the following morning from Manchester to Barcelona, so it was going to be a double wedding weekend in different countries. But when we heard that the egg collection was going to be on the Monday, we knew it just wasn't possible to make the Spanish wedding. I was devastated. But my friend who was getting married in Spain was very understanding – and now our children play together.

For anyone trying to get pregnant, whether that's naturally or through fertility treatment, the process can be challenging. From my own experience and from talking to experts, it's key to keep communicating with your partner or confidante, and the clinic that you choose, as well as ensuring you take the pressure off your mind and body. Just remember to give yourself a break. Be kind to yourself! After all, we're only human – no one makes the right decisions all the time and no one's body is perfect.

'The whole thing felt pretty stressful. We tried to stay optimistic but overall it felt quite draining. We definitely had our share of heated arguments! But it made our relationship stronger at times. We ended up treating IVF like something that just needed to be done, it was much easier not talking or thinking about it too much. We distracted ourselves with other things.' **SOPHIE**

'I felt my relationship with my wife was good during the whole process. We were both in it together, focused on the process and I think I supported her well at each stage. Although it was difficult, I tried not to think too far ahead, and just focus on the next step in the process. It may have put a strain on us if we had to go through multiple cycles.' **VENKI**

## Stripping the romance out of sex

Sex can be a fairly taboo subject. You may well never have discussed your sexual relationship with anyone before – maybe not even with your partner. Sex may just be something that bonds you physically and emotionally, it could not be something that is up for discussion.

So, when you first enter the IVF world, you may well feel embarrassed by having to reveal so much about yourself – your personal life, your reproductive health, your relationship... From my experience, this embarrassment quickly disappears. The consultants, nurses and counsellors at your clinic are professionals and should make you feel comfortable with discussing intimate details. You will probably find that you become very pragmatic about the whole process.

Of course, IVF is a clinical procedure that completely strips any romance out of sex. Not that you're likely to feel that up to it anyway, with your hormones all over the place from the drugs and your body feeling slightly sore from procedures.

It's worth remembering that, for many couples, trying for a baby naturally may still involve some planning and relatively unromantic sex. Indeed, one friend once told me that they organised their sex life into 'fun sex' and 'get-me-pregnant sex'. (Thank goodness I never had to do that. I know for a fact that Max wouldn't have appreciated such a schedule!) So, once you go down the IVF route, you may find that it takes the pressure off your sex life.

'Through the whole process I felt really depressed at points. And our relationship had its ups and downs. We got through it but I wasn't sure we would at many points. The pressure from start to finish was pretty significant. I coped by having private counselling, doing exercise, and talking to my wife. I'm now really happy we went through it, as I have two wonderful children, but I'm still fairly scarred from the ▶

whole process. My advice would be stick with it. It's tough but worth it. Try to talk lots with your partner and understand how each other is feeling.' **ANON**

'My relationship was definitely strained, especially during the treatment and injections process.' **ED**

'My husband and I feel like a team. I know exactly how he feels, he knows how I feel. We've got that bond.' **ALANA**

# Where to get help

## HFEA
The Human Fertilisation and Embryology Authority is the government's independent regulator that oversees fertility treatment and research.
www.hfea.gov.uk

## Fertility Network UK
National charity for people who experience fertility problems.
fertilitynetworkuk.org

## Your clinic
All clinics licensed by the HFEA have to offer you counselling before you start treatment. Some clinics will offer it for free, while others may require payment.

## British Infertility Counselling Association
A directory of accredited private therapists, some of whom also provide telephone and video counselling.
www.bica.net

## British Association for Counselling and Psychotherapy
www.bacp.co.uk

## Genetic Alliance
Represents different charities that support people with various genetic conditions.
www.geneticalliance.org.uk

## Daisy Network
A charity for women with premature ovarian insufficiency (POI).
www.daisynetwork.org

## www.facebook.com/groups/mensfertilitysupport/
A closed Facebook group for men (only) going through fertility treatment, which you have to request to join.

## CHAPTER 3

# How to choose a clinic

## The factors you need to consider

Once you've decided to go down the fertility treatment route, choosing a clinic can be challenging, as there are often so many options. It's hard to know where to start and who to trust. It is also a really personal decision, as everyone's situation is different and so the criteria that are important to you will depend on your circumstances.

Some patients will be eligible for NHS funding (*see* box below). If you are going private, then it's worth visiting a number of clinics before you decide where to go for treatment – go along to their open days and get a feel for the clinics. Make sure you feel comfortable with all the staff, from the receptionists right the way through to the consultants.

## NHS funding

Depending on your situation, you may be eligible for free fertility treatment on the NHS (*see* page 113). If it seems that you might be eligible for NHS funding, your GP will refer you on to a clinic that deals with NHS patients. The clinic will then determine whether you are eligible, according to various factors, such as your health.

If you are eligible for NHS funding, you may have a choice of a number of clinics – but that can depend on where you live, so in some cases you may not be able to choose your clinic. ▷

NHS-funded patients can be treated at a public hospital if it has a fertility treatment department. Some private clinics also treat patients with NHS funding. You should receive the same level of care whether you're NHS-funded or paying privately. But some private clinics taking NHS-funded patients will offer everything for free, while others offer basic IVF for free but then require 'top-up' fees for extras, such as time-lapse imaging (*see* page 122). As the basic process is the same for NHS-funded patients as for private patients, there is no difference in success rates, like for like. If the free cycle(s) of IVF isn't successful, and you decide to go private, then either you can stay on at the same clinic or transfer to a different clinic of your choice. There will be no need to do more tests, as your notes can transfer with you.

**When making your decision, there are important factors to consider:**

- Success rates
- Costs
- Services offered
- Treatment eligibility
- Location and opening hours
- Waiting times
- Inspection and patient ratings
- Add-ons offered
- Home or abroad

To help you decide which clinic might be right for you, the Human Fertilisation and Embryology Authority (HFEA) have created a clinic search section on their website, which uses all the same measures to compare different clinics around the country. The HFEA suggests visiting this website before looking at the websites of specific clinics, as each one uses different measures for their data and success rates, and so it's hard to compare like for like.

Around 80 per cent of clinics in the UK have been given a four-year licence, which indicates that overall they comply well to the standards set by the HFEA.

Dr Valentine says...

'Nobody can guarantee someone's going to get pregnant and have a baby. That is like selling get-rich-quick schemes. You've got to be realistic. What you can do is guarantee that you'll be giving them a better chance than where they start off.'

## SUCCESS RATES

With the aim being to get pregnant, people often focus on clinic success rates. But the HFEA advises against becoming too obsessed about birth rates. The authority points out that the average birth rate at a clinic won't reveal how likely you are to have a baby there. Everybody's body and circumstances are different. You'll get a better idea of your chances from speaking to a consultant.

So, when you start looking around for where to have your treatment, the key is not to get hung up on small differences in success rates between clinics. Instead, compare them with the national average, the reason being that in small clinics the success rate can be skewed by chance. For example, if a small clinic achieves a couple less births in a year, their annual success rate will drop more significantly than if the same happened at a big clinic. So, on their website, the HFEA have devised a 'reliability range' – the clinic's real birth rate performance lies somewhere within that range.

## COSTS

Back in 2013, IVF pioneer Professor Robert Winston told *The Guardian* that he was worried about the charges patients face in many clinics: 'The biggest change has been the increasingly commercial market which has driven IVF. I think that the inequalities in treatment are scandalous, and I do feel very angry that the NHS has used IVF as a money-spinner. We have a situation where your chances of having NHS-funded fertility treatment depend entirely on where you live, leaving many people unable to get the help that they need.'

Things have moved on since then. But even today, around 60 per cent of patients are having to pay for their treatment. In the UK, the average cost of one cycle of IVF is around £5000, although this varies enormously. And what starts out as a few thousand can quickly escalate when extra costs are added.

### Jheni's story…

On our second cycle of IVF at the Bristol Centre for Reproductive Medicine (BCRM), we were offered a higher dose of the egg-boosting drug Menopur. When we went through it first time round, my daily dose was 300iu, as that is what the NHS deem the maximal effective clinical dose. When we tried for our second child, we had to pay for treatment. Private patients can have more than 300iu of Menopur. Due to my low ovarian reserve, second time round our consultant, Dr Chandra, advised us to try bumping it up to 450iu. He was very clear that the stats didn't show any difference in pregnancy success rates, but he said it was worth giving it a go – if we were prepared to spend on the extra drugs. He was absolutely right to try. For the first cycle my ovaries hadn't reacted as well and he only managed to extract four eggs, all of which fertilised, but ▷

only one made it through to being a high-quality blastocyst – my daughter. Second time round, the extra drugs boosted my ovaries and we managed to get 15 eggs out – 11 fertilised, and eventually two of them became good-quality blastocysts, so one was implanted and the other put aside into the freezer.

So, despite the stats claiming there was no difference in success rates, maybe we simply got lucky or maybe Dr Chandra's experience paid off. He's been working in the field for almost two decades and so he had an inkling that it was worth a try.

Patients are often tempted to take extra drugs or try extra treatments in the hope that they might just help. It's completely understandable. When Dr Chandra told us that increasing our dose of the egg-boosting drug might increase the number of eggs, we didn't take long to mull over whether it was worth spending the extra few hundred quid it would cost us.

Extra treatment is fine if you've got the spare cash and it's a safe treatment. But some so-called add-ons being offered at clinics aren't necessarily backed up by science – or are yet to be well researched (*see* page 127).

In 2018, YouGov conducted a survey of IVF patients for the HFEA. It found that 62 per cent of patients treated at private clinics hadn't expected to pay as much as they did, although just over three-quarters (77 per cent) of patients who had add-ons were satisfied with how open and transparent the costs of these were.

So, before deciding on a clinic, make sure you have an in-depth discussion about exactly what costs are involved. It might be worth looking into clinics that offer payment packages or money-back guarantees if IVF doesn't work (generally only offered to patients who would already be considered ideal candidates for IVF). But just be absolutely sure what you're signing up to and what you will actually get for your money.

## Example of costs

A breakdown of private treatment fees (as of 2020) at the Bristol Centre for Reproductive Medicine (BCRM) where Max and I paid for our second cycle of IVF:

**First consultation**: £250 / £175 (dependent on consultant)

**Follow-up consultation:** £150 / £90 (dependent on consultant)

**Embryologist consultation:** £100

**Treatment support session with counsellor:** £50

**Diagnostic or pregnancy ultrasound scan:** £150

**Fertility MOT (couple):** £450 (comprehensive consultation including ultrasound scan, blood tests and semen analysis)

**Semen analysis:** £90 (detailed), £150 (advanced)

**IVF**: £3595 (includes patient information meeting; individual nurse planning consultation; monitoring ultrasound scans; HFEA fee; egg collection with anaesthetic sedation in the care of a consultant anaesthetist; laboratory costs; sperm preparation; assisted hatching; blastocyst/embryo culture; embryo glue if appropriate; embryo/blastocyst transfer; pregnancy scan or follow up consultation; treatment support sessions including counselling)

**Intra-Cytoplasmic Sperm Injection procedure – ICSI + IVF (as above)** : £4495

**Medication per IVF / ICSI:** £500–£1800 (approx)

**IUI**: £695 (no medication used) / £800 (excludes medication)

Donor sperm: £900 per cycle (anonymous donor) / £2035 (known donor, includes screening and storage for 1 year)

**Donor egg treatment IVF** – egg recipient cycle (includes donor eggs from unknown donor, excludes drugs and ICSI if required): £7500

**Frozen embryo transfer**: £1595 (excludes medication)

**Embryo freezing**: £495 (includes egg collection, fertilisation of eggs with sperm and embryo culture (IVF), vitrification and storage of embryos for up to 1 year)

**Embryo storage:** £295 for 1 year

**Egg freezing:** £2800 (includes egg collection, vitrification and freeze storage for up to 1 year (excludes medication)

**Sperm freezing:** £495 (includes short consultation; analysis recovery test, freeze and storage for up to 1 year)

'We raised the money for IVF by moving house, using savings and working very hard.' **NICKY**

Jessica Hepburn, author of *The Pursuit of Motherhood*, *21 Miles* and founder of Fertility Fest, says…

'I totted up how much I'd spent on IVF. I think it was about £70,000 in total. But I don't regret it.'

Paul Wilson, BCRM Head of Embryology and Andrology, says…

'IVF is very labour intensive and carried out by highly skilled staff. "Highly skilled" usually means expensive. All the products we use are expensive too and everything must be tested for toxicity. For example, we have to use sample dishes/tubes made of very high-quality plastic, which have been tested to the nth degree to show that they don't leach chemicals which have an effect on the sperm, eggs or embryos. Material and equipment prices are significant and continue to rise. Additionally, because of the restrictions on funding for training, the number of embryologists being trained has dropped in recent years, resulting in an upward pressure on the salaries of qualified staff. People are desperate to be embryologists, competition is fierce for the limited number of training posts, but the main way to become an embryologist ▷

these days is through the NHS scientist training programme, and trainee numbers in recent years have been largely dependent on funding from central government. Previously, staff were trained at each centre in conjunction with our professional body, which was more flexible and cheaper overall.'

## SERVICES OFFERED

If you've had tests at your local GP surgery and already know the fertility issue you're dealing with, then it's important to check whether the clinic offers the right treatment for you. Or you may not know what the issue is, but it's still worth looking into what services are on offer to be sure you feel confident that the clinic is right for you. For example, you might be looking for counselling to be available to help you before, during or after treatment, and not all clinics offer this at all stages. And it's also worth finding out how many cycles the clinic will attempt before trying another method or stopping treatment altogether.

Dr Valentine says...

'Top clinics will look to personalise treatment rather than generalise treatment like a production line.'

'My wife was offered counselling, but I wasn't. I felt secondary to it all really. And I felt depressed and hopeless. The longer it went on, the more we had to prepare for not having children, which was an awful thought, particularly when family had always been our dream.' **NICKY**

## TREATMENT ELIGIBILITY

Even if you're paying privately for treatment, some clinics may have specific criteria that you must meet, such as being a certain age or having a body mass index (BMI) within a certain range.

If you're eligible for NHS funding, it's worth knowing about the current system. According to current NICE guidelines for England and Wales, couples who have been trying to get pregnant for over two years, where the woman is under 40, should be offered three full cycles of NHS-funded IVF or ICSI. (If the woman turns 40 while undergoing treatment, that cycle can be completed but no further cycles offered.)

However, do bear in mind that although NICE make all these recommendations, the individual NHS clinical commissioning groups (CCGs) have the final say about who can be NHS-funded. So the local CCG criteria where you live may be stricter than the NICE recommendations. This is evident by the disparity in NHS-funded cycles between different countries in the UK. In the last decade, there has been a general trend for increased funding in Scotland. In 2018, 60 per cent of treatments were NHS funded in Scotland. In Northern Ireland 45 per cent were funded by the NHS. Meanwhile, funding in Wales has fluctuated over the last 10 years, but is now on the rise – 41 per cent of treatments were funded in 2018. But funding in England has slightly declined in the last decade, down to around 35 per cent in 2018.

NICE recommends three cycles because research published in 2017 found that more cycles of IVF led to higher success rates. The study was carried out on more than 56,000 women from Australia and New Zealand who had undergone IVF. The results showed that 33 per cent got pregnant after just one round, but by the eighth cycle the success rate was between 54 and 77 per cent. While the NHS can't afford to support eight cycles of IVF per patient, this study goes to show how, with each subsequent round of IVF, doctors learn more about how a patient's body responds to treatment, such as different doses of drugs.

The same recommendation goes for women aged between 40 and 42, but NICE suggests that they should only be offered one full cycle – and that is provided they have never had IVF before and don't suffer from a low ovarian reserve (not having many eggs).

For female same-sex couples, NICE guidelines recommend that, after six unsuccessful cycles of donor insemination, they should be offered six cycles of IUI before IVF is considered.

A worrying trend is that there has been a steady decline in NHS funding for donor insemination treatments – from 17 per cent of treatments in 2015 to 12 per cent in 2017. This impacts female same-sex couples or patients with no partner, as they need a sperm donor in order to get pregnant.

### The IVF 'postcode lottery'

The discrepancy between clinical commissioning groups (CCGs) has led to a so-called postcode lottery in England – where you live affects the number of cycles you are offered free on the NHS.

For example, at the time this book was printed, in Bristol patients receive only one free NHS-funded cycle of IVF, whereas you get three cycles for free if you live in Tameside and Glossop. There are other areas in the country where you also get three full cycles, but the criteria (such as age) are slightly more restrictive.

To highlight these differences, in 2017 the charity Fertility Fairness drew up a sort of IVF league table, ranking the NHS CCGs in different parts of England.

A report by NICE in 2018 revealed that the number of CCGs offering the recommended three IVF cycles to women under 40 had halved in the previous five years – 12 per cent of medical centres offered the three cycles compared to 24 per cent in 2013. Looking at the stats on a map reveals a big difference between the north and south – more cycles tend to be offered by CCGs in the north of England. The situation gets even more ridiculous when access to NHS funding varies for different patients attending the same clinic, because their home or their GP surgeries are in different postcodes.

This IVF postcode lottery only exists in England. In Scotland, Wales and Northern Ireland, IVF eligibility is standardised. Currently, in Scotland an eligible female partner can receive three free cycles if under 40 and one cycle between the ages of 40 and 42; in Wales it's two cycles for women under 40 and one cycle if aged between 40 and 42, and in Northern Ireland it's just one cycle for those under 40.

There have been calls to end the IVF postcode lottery in England, but for the moment it's maybe no surprise that hopeful parents-to-be are bearing it in mind if moving house. I heard of one couple who moved back from abroad and scouted around Greater London for the best borough to settle in, according to how many free cycles they would receive. Another couple ensured they kept their main address in a town where the NHS paid for three cycles of IVF, despite having to move to work in another nearby town. The whole thing is reminiscent of the school-catchment-area shenanigans, where people have been known to rent homes in a certain area in order to get their kids into the state school of their choice.

The reality is that with budgets being slashed, the NHS is having to make some tough decisions about where to make savings. The flip side is that patients may push to implant more than one embryo at the same time (see below) if only one free cycle of IVF is available.

## MULTIPLE BIRTHS

For most women, transferring one single embryo is just as successful as transferring two (*see* page 86). And it's also worth bearing in mind that multiple births (twins, triplets or more) are the single greatest health risk to both mothers and babies. There is a higher risk of miscarriage and twins are six times more likely to need neonatal care. The mother is also more likely to suffer from high blood pressure, anaemia and haemorrhaging and, while it's highly unlikely, the risk of the mother dying during childbirth is 2.5 times higher than average.

The HFEA campaign to reduce multiple births has been successful – multiple birth rate following IVF treatment is now at 8 per cent. The authority recommends finding a clinic that has a low multiple birth rate but a high success rate, to ensure you have as safe and healthy a pregnancy as possible.

## LOCATION AND OPENING HOURS

If you're embarking on IVF, you will no doubt be surprised by what is involved in undergoing treatment – such as numerous tests and consultations. Choosing a clinic that is local to where you live or work can remove the burden of having to travel long distances. If you do end up deciding on a clinic that's not close by then it's worth finding out if there are some tests that you can do at a local hospital. And check out the clinic opening hours – if they're open early or late it might help you fit in appointments around a busy work schedule.

'For our first cycle of IVF we were effectively pushed through from the NHS gynaecology department into their affiliated clinic at the same hospital, with little or no thought. After the first round failed, realising we could have more of a choice, we picked a new clinic. After ruling out a few based on online reviews, we picked the one that was most convenient to get to for regular appointments. During the first round, I had found it very stressful having to duck out of work and travel across town for (lots of!) appointments, so choosing a new location near work made a huge difference.' SOPHIE

'After our first cycle failed, the clinic we chose was local and convenient to get to, and had good results online. We knew we would have to go to the clinic often, so it was important to limit the stress and hassle of attending appointments while also managing busy jobs.' ED

## WAITING TIMES

If time is against you, maybe because of age, or because you're due for treatment/surgery for another condition, you may not want to wait around for a fertility clinic to have a space for you. So it's worth finding out how long you'll have to wait before the clinic can start treatment – particularly if you're using donor eggs, sperm or embryos, which can involve waiting a long time for them to become available. (More on this in chapter 4.)

## INSPECTION AND PATIENT RATINGS

Clinics can't operate in the UK unless they have a licence from the HFEA. Inspections happen every two years, but clinics deemed to be of a good standard can be granted a licence for up to four years. The inspection assesses things such as how well eggs, sperm and embryos are stored, the standard of equipment and facilities, and whether staff are suitably qualified. On their website, the HFEA lists every clinic's inspection rating, as well as patient ratings, where patients comment on things like how caring the staff are, how easy it is to book an appointment, or whether they ended up paying what they expected at the start.

At an open day or clinic visit, get a feel for it and how the staff treat you. Make sure you ask lots of questions, and chat to other patients if possible.

## ADD-ONS

Add-ons are optional additional treatments that you can have on top of standard IVF or ICSI. Some of these extras are techniques that have existed for a while but have never been proven to improve birth rates, while others are newer techniques that initial studies have shown to be beneficial but more research is needed.

When you see studies reported, you don't always have the whole picture. A clinic might offer an add-on that they believe improves their success rates, but the science doesn't back it up. Or maybe a newspaper reports an incredible new treatment that is going to revolutionise IVF, but it's reporting a talk that someone has just given at a conference, as opposed to an academic paper that has been peer reviewed. So it's important to determine where the evidence is coming from, how large a group has been studied, and what exactly has been achieved – a higher pregnancy rate or a higher live birth rate?

The most rigorous type of test that gives the best evidence is from something called a randomised controlled trial (RCT), where scientists randomly assign patients to two different groups. One half are given the treatment being tested, and the other half (the control group) are given a conventional treatment or a placebo. Then you compare the outcomes. The larger the RCT, the more meaningful the evidence. A systematic review of a number of RCTs will give a really valuable result.

To help you decide which add-ons are worth investing in and which are not, the HFEA have a 'traffic light' rating system for them on their website. The authority awards a green light to add-ons where there is evidence of more than one good-quality RCT, proving the treatment is effective and, crucially, safe. An amber light is given to treatments where there is little or conflicting evidence, and a red light is given if there is no evidence. However, at the moment, no add-ons have been given the green light. It's important to note that amber light treatment may be beneficial, but not enough research has been carried out to confirm this.

Some clinics will offer some add-ons as part of the treatment, others will charge extra for some or all of them. If you're being funded by the NHS, you won't have add-ons included in your treatment unless the clinic does it as standard. If you're paying privately, it may surprise you that the cost of certain add-ons can vary hugely between clinics. For example, an endometrial scratch (*see* page 120) can range in price from being just over £100 to several hundred, depending on the clinic.

So, before signing up to any add-on, make sure you discuss with your consultant why the treatment might work for you personally, such as if they've seen success with other patients, and whether the cost compares favourably to other clinics, and then weigh up whether you can afford it. If you have a load of add-ons, you might find that you end up spending almost as much on all of these as you're paying for the actual IVF, and then don't have enough money to pay for more treatment cycles if needed.

'Each round of IVF we had more and more add-ons – glue, hatching, scratch, my wife took three kinds of progesterone, and we had a delayed cycle the final time.' NICKY

## ASSISTED HATCHING

This is exactly what it sounds like – the embryo is helped to 'hatch' using an acidic solution, lasers or other tools to thin or pierce the thick layer that surrounds the embryo. The technique was developed as some experts believe implantation rates are higher for embryos with a thin membrane. It is thought that this membrane may be thicker in some older women, and so thinning it may help the embryos to hatch. But more research is needed, and there is a risk that the embryo could become damaged in the process.

Currently, NICE says: 'Assisted hatching is not recommended because it has not been shown to improve pregnancy rates.' NICE also says more research is needed into the effects on babies born as a result of assisted hatching. So the HFEA has given assisted hatching a red light, according to their traffic-light rating system.

Paul Wilson says...

'When we looked at our data historically, going back to when we first started to offer assisted hatching, which I think was 1999, we found that when we introduced it, we seemed to see a jump in success rates. Not huge jumps, but steps in the right direction. However, as our systems have developed it has become harder to see a benefit of hatching, so we are now no longer comfortable charging money for it. We can carry out hatching very safely, so we're happy to offer it free of charge for the groups that we believe may possibly benefit, but the potential benefit has to outweigh the potential risks.'

## ENDOMETRIAL SCRATCH

Embryos need to implant in the wall of the uterus, known as the endometrium. Estimates suggest that up to 85 per cent of embryos do not implant, and implantation rate per embryo transfer is 10–15 per cent if they're implanted on day 2 or 3 of treatment, and 23–25 per cent for blastocyst transfers (on day 5 or 6). Sometimes implantation doesn't occur because they're not fully developed or the endometrium isn't at the right stage of development when the embryo tries to implant. But occasionally, it's because the endometrium isn't fit to receive an embryo.

The idea behind this technique is that scraping the endometrium with a sterile plastic tube before embryo transfer causes the body to release chemicals and hormones to repair the scratch site, hence creating the right environment for the embryo to implant into. But there is a slight risk of infection. And at the moment only a few, moderate-quality studies have been carried out, so the HFEA has given this technique an amber light in their rating system. However, there are some more large-scale studies currently taking place.

## EMBRYO GLUE

The active substance in the glue is something called hyaluronan. Before embryo transfer, the glue is added to the solution in the dish containing the embryo, which may improve the chance of it implanting. There aren't any known risks. Despite one high-quality study showing a 10 per cent increase in pregnancy and birth rates, which is backed up by a few other studies of moderate quality, the HFEA has given the technique an amber light rating, as they feel more research is needed.

Paul Wilson says...

'The problem is that randomised controlled trials [RCTs], where high-quality evidence is obtained, are incredibly expensive and complex to run and therefore beyond the resources of most individual clinics or the NHS. That's when it starts to become a problem, because [the clinic has] got some evidence of benefit, but it's not necessarily high-quality evidence, so we're then faced with the dilemma of whether we offer the add-on or not, particularly if other clinical groups or the published literature also reports or suggests a benefit.

## ELECTIVE FREEZING

Usually when you go through IVF or ICSI, an embryo is transferred to the uterus a few days after fertilisation in what is known as a 'fresh cycle', and any spare embryos are frozen for future use. But some patients decide before they even start treatment that after the fertilisation stage they will definitely freeze all embryos and store them for a few weeks or months, before transferring to the uterus at a later date. This means that no embryos are transferred in the fresh cycle.

The logic behind this is that some research has shown that the endometrium can be affected by fertility drugs, and so waiting a few months gives your body the chance to flush them out of your system. Some evidence also suggests that babies born from frozen embryos are closer in birth weight to naturally conceived babies, as babies from fresh cycle IVF have been known to have a lower birth weight, which can affect health later on.

There's always a risk that an embryo might not survive the thawing process. But it's becoming more and more popular – in the US, around a quarter of IVF cycles now use this strategy.

Currently, there's a lot of discussion around elective freezing. So far, the HFEA has given it an amber light rating. This is because experts aren't sure yet whether freeze-all cycles are more effective. The most recent research suggested no benefit. Published in 2019, the study of 460 women at clinics in Denmark, Sweden and Spain showed a tiny difference in success rates – 26 per cent for freeze-all cycles versus 29 per cent for one embryo transferred on fresh cycle. But a large-scale clinical trial called E-Freeze is happening at the moment, which should hopefully help to clarify the debate.

## TIME-LAPSE IMAGING

In standard IVF or ICSI, every day the embryologist briefly removes the dish containing the embryos from the incubator to check on their development. Some experts think this may interfere with embryo development. In a time-lapse system, the embryos don't need to be removed from the incubator, as cameras in the time-lapse imaging machine allow the embryologist to capture thousands of images of the embryos as they develop, without disturbing them. So the embryologist gets a constant view of the embryos and can check on them at any time during their development. A time-lapse imaging system can also apply software to help the embryologist choose the best-quality embryo at the optimum time.

There are no known risks. A 2019 review of a number of different studies found no good evidence that time-lapse imaging is more or less effective than conventional methods. Indeed, the HFEA has given it an amber light rating, as there is currently not enough evidence to show it improves birth rates. But the authority recognises the technique has potential and more research is needed.

Paul Wilson says…

'Traditionally, we would take the dish containing the embryos out of the incubator once or twice a day to assess the embryos. It's rather like taking a photograph and you're making judgements based on what you see at that specific moment in time. Furthermore, when we take the embryos out, we're exposing them to air, light, temperature changes and so on. Time-lapse incubation means the embryo isn't exposed to those changes, as the incubators allow us to take a picture of the embryos using a high-powered microscope built into the machine every 10 or 15 minutes, 24 hours a day. We can then string the images together to create a video of development. Additionally, we can mark certain time-points in embryo development and create models which may help us to say: "The embryo development pattern here most closely matches one that led to a pregnancy for another patient, so that's the embryo we should transfer." We may also be able to use these models to assign scores to embryos and, in doing so, potentially rank them in order of quality and/or implantation potential.'

## PRE-IMPLANTATION GENETIC SCREENING (PGS)

Chromosomes are the structures inside cells that carry genes and are mostly made of DNA. Females usually have two X chromosomes (XX) and males have one X and one Y (XY). Sometimes embryos develop with an abnormal number of chromosomes. These 'aneuploid embryos' may not develop into a baby, or may lead to a baby with a genetic condition.

Pre-implantation genetic screening (PGS) is a technique that tests embryos to see if they have the normal number of chromosomes. It involves removing a cell or a few cells from the embryo to analyse them for chromosomal abnormalities. An embryo with the normal number of chromosomes can then be transferred to the uterus.

While the removal of the cell(s) shouldn't affect the embryo development, occasionally there are some risks with this technique: removing the cell(s) could damage the embryo, mean a healthy embryo has to be discarded, or it could cause problems in foetal development. There is also a chance that PGS won't spot a problem, as the tested cell may differ from the others in the embryo.

The HFEA has given PGS a red light rating, because some studies have shown that it decreases success rates, possibly due to damage to the embryo. It's worth bearing this in mind if you're offered PGS by your clinic. Plus, it can be really expensive.

PGS should not be confused with PGD (*see* pages 83 and 215).

## INTRACYTOPLASMIC MORPHOLOGIC SPERM INJECTION (IMSI)

This technique involves selecting the best sperm for ICSI, based on how they look. The embryologist inspects the sperm under a very powerful microscope. There are no extra risks, but the HFEA has given it a red light rating, as the evidence is still minimal as to whether it really improves success rates – one review showed it might help if

ICSI had failed before, and another small study suggested it might be beneficial for men whose partners were older.

## PHYSIOLOGICAL INTRACYTOPLASMIC SPERM INJECTION (PICSI)

This technique is also about selecting the best sperm for ICSI, but it involves putting sperm in a solution of hyaluronic acid (HA) – a natural compound found in the body – and analysing which ones bind to the HA. The sperm that bind well are then used for ICSI. PICSI has been given a red light rating by the HFEA, as studies haven't shown any difference in success rates between the technique and just doing ICSI.

## ARTIFICIAL EGG ACTIVATION

Egg activation takes place when a sperm meets an egg, triggering embryo development and preventing other sperm from fertilising the egg. So-called calcium ionophores can be added to the Petri dish containing the egg and sperm to stimulate this process.

A few studies have shown the treatment may improve success rates, but there are concerns over the risks. Some experts think that the treatment might cause embryos to develop with abnormal numbers of chromosomes – aneuploid embryos. So clinics should only offer this treatment to certain patients which they feel will benefit. Make sure you ask why if you're offered artificial egg activation. The HFEA has given it an amber light rating.

## INTRAUTERINE CULTURE

In standard IVF or ICSI, embryos develop in a fluid in an incubator. Intrauterine culture involves the egg being fertilised and placed in a device inserted into the mother's uterus for a few hours during early embryo development. While it might seem like a good idea for the embryo to initially develop in the natural environment, this part of the process would in fact normally occur in the fallopian tubes, so critics question whether there is any benefit to this procedure. And there's no evidence that this technique is beneficial or safe. So it's probably not worth the extra cost. The HFEA has given it a red light rating.

## REPRODUCTIVE IMMUNOLOGY TESTS

Some experts believe that some cases of infertility or miscarriage may be caused by the mother's immune system rejecting the embryo, as it has different 'genetic variants'. For example, natural killer cells are a type of white blood cell that help fight things like infection and tumours. As uterine natural killer (uNK) cells are a major part of the white blood cell population in the endometrium at the time of implantation, recently they have received a lot of attention as to their role in normal implantation and early placental development. But there is no convincing evidence that a woman's immune system won't accept an embryo because of differences in genetic variants. Quite the opposite – experts have found that the embryo and mother's immune system work together. If you think about it, the immune system will have evolved so that it accepts an embryo with different DNA, because roughly half of its variants will have differences because they come from the father.

The HFEA has given reproductive immunology tests and treatment a red light rating, and warn against treatments to suppress the immune system as there are risks involved. For example, taking steroids can cause high blood pressure, diabetes and premature birth. Meanwhile, intravenous immunoglobulins (IVIg) can cause side effects such as headaches, muscle pain, fever, chills, low back pain, and occasionally blood clots, kidney failure and anaphylaxis. And intralipid infusions can also cause headaches, as well as dizziness, flushing, nausea and sometimes clotting or infection.

It's important to remember that the vast majority of healthcare professionals have only your best interests at heart – and would only recommend a certain add-on if they felt it could be beneficial. Indeed, we grow up putting our trust in medical professionals – and rightly so. However, the fertility industry is becoming increasingly commercialised. Take the case of the clinics offering money-back schemes (generally only offered to patients who would already be considered ideal candidates for IVF). Or how about the story where a couple won a cycle of IVF (it worked, they've now got a baby)? The industry is certainly evolving for commercial interests.

## PROFITS BEFORE PATIENTS

In recent years, a few unscrupulous clinics have been criticised for taking advantage of vulnerable patients who are desperate to have a baby. In 2019, the BMJ published a statement from the HFEA and 10 leading professional and patient fertility groups expressing concerns that patients are often being offered and paying for add-ons that claim to improve their chances of having a healthy baby when there is currently insufficient evidence. In some cases, clinics are charging up to four times as much as is reasonable for IVF treatment, because of the cost of all the add-ons.

'A cycle shouldn't cost more than £5000 – £3000 to £4000 plus an extra £1000 maybe for an extra frozen embryo transfer,' the HFEA chair Sally Cheshire told *The Telegraph* in an interview in 2019. 'Yet we hear anecdotal evidence of cycles which are £10,000, £15,000 or even £20,000. We have no legal powers to regulate prices. I would love the [1991 Human Fertilisation and Embryology Act] to change ... to give us economic powers of regulation.'

Other clinics have been criticised for selectively reporting success rates, or using aggressive sales tactics to target older women while not being honest about the true odds of them getting pregnant.

In 2017, in the UK, 10,835 women over 40 had IVF, but only 75 of them aged 42 to 43 had a baby using their own eggs. And between 2004 and 2017, the success rate for women over the age of 44 was just 1 per cent.

'What the clinics shouldn't be doing is trading on hope and vulnerability,' said Cheshire. 'They should be honest and transparent about a woman or a couple's chances. We need to be doing the right thing by our patients – making sure that the price is not exploitative; that the information is accurate and that patients are not being offered add-on treatments that are unproven without the facts.'

In general, UK clinics are highly ethical and have their patients' best interests at heart. And in the UK, we're lucky that we have the HFEA to regulate the fertility industry. But it's always worth asking a clinic a lot of questions before signing up to treatment to be sure that you're comfortable with the facility, the staff, the type of treatment, add-ons and other services you're being offered, as well as being clear on the costs.

## GOING ABROAD FOR TREATMENT

IVF can be expensive and donor waiting lists long in the UK, so more of us are looking into having treatment abroad, because it can be a quicker, cheaper option. However, at the time of printing, we're still unsure whether Brexit will have an effect.

The HFEA recommend doing in-depth research and looking into options in the UK first before enquiring abroad. Treatment in the UK may not end up being any more expensive when you factor in all the extras involved in going abroad, such as flights, hotels, specialist medical insurance, unpaid leave. And if you're looking abroad because you think the wait might be too long in the UK, you may find that donor egg waiting lists in this country are not as long as you imagine (*see* 'Where to get help' on page 137).

If you do decide to look into treatment abroad, it's important to remember that foreign clinics aren't necessarily regulated in the same way that they are in this country. Some nations have governing bodies, like the HFEA, that license clinics and oversee fertility treatments. But many countries do not. So it's worth enquiring about a national regulator when researching a clinic. And bear in mind that, although the EU does have certain standards on quality and safety, some countries in the EU are not adhering to legislation. The HFEA has no influence overseas to help you if something goes wrong. If you have any doubts, it might be worth getting legal advice (*see* 'Where to get help' on page 137).

## SUCCESS RATES ABROAD

Clinics abroad can seem like they have incredible success rates. But just be aware that they may be selective in the data they are publishing. For example, they could be reporting their pregnancy rates as opposed to live birth rates, or only showing data for women under a certain age.

## YOUR SITUATION

Some countries don't offer treatment to single women or same-sex couples, so check this out first before doing too much research on one particular clinic.

### Sex selection

Pre-implantation genetic diagnosis (PGD) or pre-implantation genetic testing (PGT-M) is a technique used to analyse the genetic make-up of an embryo (*see* page 215).

In the UK, PGD is only used to screen for genes linked to serious genetic conditions. It is illegal for sex selection – as is the case in ▶

much of the world. But sex selection using PGD *is* legal in the US, where some clinics offer it to help with 'family balancing' – in other words, for families who have children of one particular sex and who would like to add to their family with a child of the opposite sex. But there are reports that it is being used by first-time parents, keen to have a child of a particular sex. While there is no law in the US to prevent this, critics have raised concerns that it could have societal implications, particularly in countries such as China or India, where some families have a preference for boys.

## DONOR LAW ABROAD

If you need a donor egg, sperm or embryo (*see* chapter 4 for more information on donation) and you're considering sourcing abroad, it's important to be aware that this can vary enormously between countries. In the UK, donors are screened for infectious diseases and serious genetic diseases, recipients know the donor family history, and donors must have counselling to ensure they recognise the importance of their decision. In the UK, the donor has no rights to the child, but from the age of 16 a donor-conceived child can find out some information about their donor through the HFEA, and from the age of 18 they can get more information, such as donor contact details. This is if the eggs or sperm were donated after 2005. Before 2005, the law ensures that donors can remain anonymous, unless they choose to have that anonymity removed.

In other countries, all this could be very different, so make sure you're happy with the donation process. Many other countries have anonymous donations. At this point in time you might think you don't want to have donor traceability. But you may change your mind and any child might want to trace back their donor.

If you've got any questions or concerns, it's worth contacting the Donor Conception Network or the National Gamete Donation Trust for advice (*see* 'Where to get help' on page 137).

Natalie Gamble, Fertility Lawyer, NGA Law, says…

'If you go to a clinic overseas [for sperm donation], you may want to get married before you go through your treatment in order to avoid having to go through an adoption process after birth. This is because if you are an unmarried couple, there is a process to go through to create legal parenthood for the second parent.'

## COSTS ABROAD

IVF can often seem cheaper when you look at a clinic website abroad. Indeed, the headline price that you see on the clinic website often seems to be very reasonable. But it's really important to be aware that the headline price is rarely what you will actually end up paying. It often doesn't include blood tests, scans, extra consultations, fertility drugs. And it's worth bearing in mind that while budget airline flights may be cheap when you book ahead, you might suddenly need to fly at short notice, when flights can be a lot more expensive.

Fertility Network UK did a survey on people who had been overseas for treatment, and one of the main criticisms they had was that it could end up being much more expensive than they'd initially thought.

Beware!

Alarm bells should sound in your head if you experience any of the following while researching a clinic abroad:

- Success rates that seem too good to be true
- Very low costs – they may not include extras for things like fertility drugs or blood tests
- High multiple pregnancy rates – multiple births are the single greatest health risk to both mothers and babies
- No limit on the number of times the same donor can donate sperm
- Reviews on clinic websites or forums that don't sound like real patients

## A BOOMING BUSINESS

In short, fertility tourism is booming. While many clinics abroad will be highly professional and trustworthy, and lots of people that go abroad for treatment are very happy with the process, there may be a few that will manipulate stats and be happy to take your hard-earned cash. And there are all sorts of extras that you can end up spending your money on, which aren't necessary. There are even IVF travel agents now!

So the main message is: make sure you do your research. Treatment and regulations vary so much between countries that it's not possible to go into the nitty-gritty of all the different scenarios here. But the website Fertility Treatment Abroad (*see* 'Where to get help' on page 137) can help with the decision process, offering useful practical information, such as popular destinations, standards and safety, legal issues and average costs.

CASE STUDY

### Ann's IVF journey to Spain

'The journey started when I had just turned 40. An early miscarriage and then months of no success led me to my GP for help. This took us down the NHS path of cycle monitoring, blood tests, laparoscopy and semen analysis, all of which proved to be normal. Another early miscarriage, two cycles on [the egg boosting drug] Clomid and yet another miscarriage could now only mean one thing... my eggs were too old. The decision had been made for us. Why waste valuable time and money trying IVF with my own eggs when it would be extremely unlikely to be successful. We would have to use donated eggs.

'We had been told from the outset that we were not entitled to any free cycles on the NHS because John had children from a previous marriage and I was over 40. However, because of our ongoing disappointing experiences at the NHS hospital we attended, we had already been considering a specialised fertility clinic. While we will always be grateful for having the tests carried out through the NHS, little filled us with confidence for the ongoing process. After researching some clinics in England, information seemed limited, success rates didn't excite us and donors were relatively sparse.

'By the time all our NHS medical tests had come to an end, we had decided to look at clinics in Spain. My husband had friends in Barcelona and loved the city so we started our search there. We found a few that looked decent, but one in particular stood out. Their website was informative: great success rates, an abundance of donors, completely set up to have patients from all around the world, established for 90 years and were at the forefront of amazing pioneering technology. On YouTube I found inspiring talks from their gynaecologists ranging from how donors were evaluated, to their ▶

latest groundbreaking technologies. The underlying message we had when researching this clinic was that they really cared about making families. The clinic filled us with confidence.

'Our first step was to arrange a video call to discuss the process and answer our many questions. Within a few days of contacting the clinic we were greeted on screen by one of their team, who was fluent in English and very knowledgeable. After the call we were relieved and happy that we had found a clinic that met all our needs and in which we had confidence even at this very early stage. We filled out all the necessary paperwork, sent off all the medical test results and the next part of our journey began.

'Four weeks later we were in Barcelona for an initial meeting. We met with our assigned gynaecologist, who explained the process in more detail and gave us several options to consider. We gave blood samples, I had a catheter test and my husband gave a semen sample. All this took just a few hours and then we were sent off with a prescription to get all the necessary tablets and pessaries needed for before and after the transfer. At this point it became clear that having had the investigative tests in the UK speeded up the process and our case could be evaluated quickly.

'We now had several decisions to make: how many embryos to transfer and at what stage, 3 or 5 days old. We decided on a 'day 5' old blastocyst and took their advice to only transfer one due to the increased risks associated with a multiple birth. We also opted to use the embryoscope [time-lapse imaging], which is an incubator in which the embryos live before transfer, but with the amazing bonus of having a camera to continuously capture shots of their growth. The great thing about this is that the embryos don't need to be removed daily to be checked, exposing them to unnatural conditions. For patients this is wonderful, because they can watch their embryos grow from being one cell old! While in the embryoscope our embryos would also have music played to them. We were told this would simulate micro vibrations which produce movement similar to those that a fertilised egg would experience in a naturally occurring pregnancy as it travelled through the fallopian tube to the uterus. This innovation was developed at the clinic and has enhanced their success rates.

'Back at home we waited patiently for news and just a few weeks later a donor and back-up donor had been matched to me, based on observable characteristics and blood type. Days later I began taking hormone supplements to start synchronising our cycles ready for the transfer of a fresh embryo.

'Having had a scan in England to check for endometrial thickness, and booked the flights and accommodation for the transfer, we received a telephone call to say the donor hadn't produced the minimum guaranteed number of eggs, so they were now preparing the back-up donor, who was a week behind in her cycle. We'd been told this might happen so we had booked flights that could be changed. At the time, this news was devastating because we were excited and ready to go, now we had to wait another week, change our travel plans, as well as now worry in case this donor also didn't produce enough eggs.

'A week later than planned we were in Barcelona. We had been advised to go over a few days early in case none of the embryos looked like they would evolve to the blastocyst stage and therefore we would have to transfer early. So with no guarantees that any of the eight eggs harvested from the donor were even going to mature into good-quality embryos, our days in Barcelona were filled with hope and excitement, but also worry. As we'd opted to use the embryoscope, we could take comfort at every opportunity by logging onto the website and watching our embryos grow. My friends and family back home also watched and helped share in the fascinating and unbelievable journey of human life. I'd researched what a good-quality blastocyst should look like and by the morning of the transfer we could see for ourselves that two were high grade and suitable for transfer.

'Sure enough, when we arrived at the clinic two were suitable and some uncertainty about a third one, which they needed to let grow to day 6 to see what happened. We had the transfer of one fresh 5-day-old blastocyst embryo and then travelled home the following day, which is when the hard work for me started; I now had to increase the hormones I was taking to every 12 hours for pessaries and 8 hours for tablets. While adjusting to this new routine was a temporary yet small price to pay, it was a worry not only remembering to take them but also the right one and at the right time; I had pessaries and tablets everywhere, in the car, in all my bags and at work. Surprisingly, though, there were only a couple of occasions when I was late taking them or I forgot. Luckily, I had a fabulous medical assistant; he was prompt at returning emails and always reassured me when I had any questions or concerns; for the many months of treatment he became an important part of my life.

'We now had the agonising two-week wait until I took the pregnancy test. Positive was an unbelievable relief, but I couldn't get excited; I now knew so much about the whole amazing life process, about everything that had to happen to keep the pregnancy ongoing, the risk factors, the possible complications. It was consuming.

'A nervous day for me was 10 weeks after the transfer when I stopped taking the hormone supplements. My medical assistant assured me that my body would now be able to do its job unaided and sure enough it did. My pregnancy continued and almost a year to the day since our first trip to the clinic I gave birth to a wonderful baby boy.

'When our treatment began at the clinic we had decided to vitrify [freeze] any embryos not transferred. Luckily, we had two; the third fresh embryo had matured to a good quality by day 6, although we were told it was less likely to implant. So two years on we tried again with a frozen embryo. Sadly, our next attempt was not successful, but we still had one left. Happily, on our last attempt our day 6 embryo progressed to a healthy pregnancy and we now have a beautiful little girl.

'Our journey has been stressful, tiring, at times devastating, and ultimately joyful. We were lucky enough to be able to give ourselves the best chances of success as the thought of having a baby which didn't have my genetic make-up never bothered me. I have always believed nurture is more important than nature. We were also lucky with our choice of clinic, not only because of their great success rates, facilities, service and staff, but because of their donor selection – I've lost count of the number of people that tell me my children look like me.'

# Where to get help

## HFEA Choose a clinic

The HFEA's useful 'Choose a clinic' service, where you can enter a postcode and hone your search options to find out details about each clinic, such as inspection ratings, patient ratings and success rates. www.hfea.gov.uk/choose-a-clinic/clinic-search

## Donor Conception Network

This is a good support network for families of donor-conceived children. If you're considering using donor eggs or sperm, it would be worth getting in touch with them: www.dcnetwork.org

## Sperm, Egg and Embryo Donation (SEED) Trust

This charity is another good source of information on donation as they are also impartial.
https://seedtrust.org.uk

## Donor recruitment agencies

If you're looking for a donor, the HFEA recommends these two agencies:
Altrui – www.altrui.co.uk
Brilliant Beginnings – www.brilliantbeginnings.co.uk

## Natalie Gamble Associates

Law firm who specialises in fertility law, family law, surrogacy, same-sex parenting and family law disputes.
www.ngalaw.co.uk

## Fertility Treatment Abroad

A website with useful practical information, such as popular destinations, standards and safety, legal issues and average costs.
https://fertility.treatmentabroad.com

## CHAPTER 4

# Egg, sperm and embryo donation

## What is involved, how to source a donor and legal issues

Every year, around 1750 babies are born in this country using donated eggs or sperm. The use of donor eggs and sperm is on the rise. Indeed, donor eggs can dramatically improve the chances of having a baby - over 25 per cent for all ages. This is because egg donors are on average five years younger than the average IVF patient. So, if you're slightly older, it might be worth considering using donor eggs.

Nina Barnsley, Director of the Donor Conception Network (DCN), says…

'The public, and even some professionals working in the fertility world, often mix up IVF and donor conception. People will just say IVF when they mean egg donation with IVF and it would be great to try to clearly differentiate treatment (for example IVF, ICSI, DI [donor insemination]) from the use of donor gametes. Single women and lesbian couples will need to use donor sperm to have a child but may not use IVF (or indeed any fertility treatment at all). A headline such as "55-year-old woman has twins after IVF" is misleading, as the key

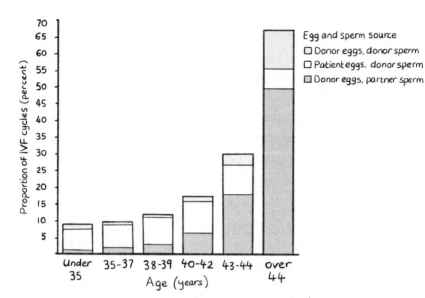

Graph shows proportion of IVF cycles using donor sperm/eggs by age band, 2018.
Source: HFEA.

| Woman's age | % of IVF cycles that resulted in a birth (per embryo transferred) |
|---|---|
| under 35 | 32.8% |
| 35 – 37 | 30.1% |
| 38 – 39 | 30.5% |
| 40 – 42 | 31.8% |
| 43 - 44 | 33.1% |
| Over 44 | 27.5% |

Success rates according to the age of egg recipient for patients using donor eggs and their partner's sperm, 2018. Source: HFEA.

element in the story is that she will almost certainly have used donor eggs for those children. It is the egg donation that made the pregnancy possible more than the IVF per se.'

Your clinic might recommend using a donor if you don't produce many (or any) eggs or sperm yourself, if their quality means they are unlikely to enable conception, or if you risk passing on an inherited disease. And if you are single or in a same-sex couple you will obviously need to use a donor, whether that is someone that you know, such as a friend, or a donor that you source through a sperm or egg bank (see page 142). If you're female and don't have fertility issues, then you may not need IVF and may just be able to have IUI.

Deciding whether to use donor eggs or sperm can be a big decision. If you're considering this then it might be worth chatting to family, friends or a counsellor to help you decide.

For people with fertility issues, donor gametes (sperm or eggs) gives them a chance at a family, but some may find it hard to consider not having their own biological baby, as maybe they had hoped to see their genes passed on and so feel a sense of loss that they won't be having their own genetic child.

But it's worth considering the role of the birth mother (the egg recipient) and something known as epigenetics – how lifestyle and the environment influences genes. For example, the birth mother will influence the so-called epigenetic marks on a baby's DNA (see box on the next page). So the environment in the uterus (womb), stress levels, diet during pregnancy and various other lifestyle factors could influence how the baby's genes are expressed. Also, if the birth mother breastfeeds, then her milk will shape the baby's immune system and gut microbiome (the genetic material of all the microbes in your intestines).

And then there is the fact that we humans are 99.9 per cent identical in terms of our DNA. So the information encoded in genes for, say, hair colour is likely to be the same. And, anyway, all our genes are inherited, so if you track far enough back, you will have the same

### Example of costs

A breakdown of some of the treatment fees involved in donation (as of 2020) at the Bristol Centre for Reproductive Medicine (BCRM):

**Use of donor sperm per cycle of treatment** (anonymous donor): £900

**Use of donor sperm** (known donor, donor screening and storage for up to 1 year): £2035

**Import of donor sperm from commercial supplier** (includes storage for up to 1 year): £195

**HFEA licence fee per insemination cycle using donor sperm (DI):** £40

**Donor egg treatment IVF** – egg recipient cycle (includes donor eggs from unknown donor, excludes drugs and ICSI if required): £7500

**Donor egg treatment IVF** – egg recipient cycle – supplement for known donor (non-refundable donor screening charge): £975
*See* page 110 for other treatment costs.

## HOW TO CHOOSE A DONOR

To help you find the right match for you, egg/sperm donation sites or egg/sperm banks will provide a lot of details about a donor, such as:

- what they look like (height, weight, eye and hair colour)
- where and when they were born
- their ethnicity
- their medical history
- if they're married or not
- if they already have any children, and if so how many and their sex

Each donor is also expected to provide a goodwill message to any children conceived.

## THE LAW

A child born from the donation of an egg, sperm or embryo will be able to apply to the HFEA for non-identifying information about the donor when they turn 16. At 18 they can get identifying information such as the donor's name, date of birth and last known address – although if the donor donated before 1 April 2005 their anonymity is protected (unless they choose to have it removed).

Donors can only find out from the HFEA the number, sex and year of birth of any children born as a result of their donation. This is to ensure that the donor can't contact the child.

Natalie Gamble, Fertility Lawyer, NGA Law, says…

'The law in relation to motherhood is simple and comes down to one rule: the person who gives birth is the legal mother, and she (or he, if transgender) is the only legal mother. It does not matter who has provided the egg – it could be a donor or perhaps the birth mother's partner or an intended mother in a surrogacy. In such cases the egg provider is not the legal mother of the child if she has not given birth.

'It gets more complicated with sperm donation. The critical date is the date of conception. Provided a couple is married or in a civil partnership at that date, and both partners consent to the artificial conception, then the spouse will be the other parent. So, if the spouse is a man, he will be the child's father. If the spouse is a woman, she will be the female second parent. There are no particular forms or processes to follow to establish that – it is just a question of the facts at the time of conception. The rules are slightly different if the intended parents are an unmarried couple – by which I mean that the birth mother is not married to or in a civil partnership with ▶

her partner. There is then a process to go through to create legal parenthood for the second parent and it only applies if the treatment takes place at a fertility clinic in the UK.

'Co-parenting and known donation arrangements do not easily fit into boxes, and the rules can be complicated. At one end of the spectrum are arrangements with a donor who is known to the parent(s), but not involved in the child's life. At the other end of the spectrum are people who share parenting fully as co-parents. But most arrangements fall somewhere in between and there is a lot of grey area. Having a written agreement will not change who the child's legal parents are, but it does enable everybody to be really clear about their intentions, so they all know what they're signing up to. We sadly do deal with cases quite frequently where things break down at a later stage, and very often they involve situations where there was always a mismatch of expectations.

'There's a whole list of reasons why having a legal connection with your child is important: being recorded on the child's birth certificate, making decisions for your child (such as where your child goes to school, whether they have medical treatment, how they're brought up, whether they move overseas, all of those sorts of ongoing parenting decisions that you make as a child grows up); your right to make court applications if you separate from your partner, your child's right to inheritance and nationality. These things can be really important further down the line.'

## BECOMING A DONOR

Donating sperm, eggs or embryos is a pretty generous thing to do – you give others a chance at having a family. But it's also a huge decision, with plenty of legal implications, and so is something to think carefully about. You won't have any legal rights or responsibilities for any children born as a result of your donation, but you will not be able to remain anonymous – unless you donated before the law changed in 2005. *See* page 144 for details.

All potential donors have to sign up to receive counselling in order to make sure that they are fully aware of the implications and the possible impact on themselves and their families. And all donors have to complete a consent form to confirm how they want their sperm, eggs or embryos to be used and stored. They can also donate eggs, sperm or embryos for use in research.

## SPERM DONATION

There are a number of ways to donate sperm. You can donate to a family member, but there are some restrictions. For example, a brother can donate sperm to his brother who has his own partner or egg donor, or a sister donate eggs to her sister. But a brother cannot donate sperm for his sister to use with her eggs, and vice versa, as they would be too genetically similar and that constitutes incest.

You can also donate to a friend. Whether you're a family member or a friend, sperm donation can either be done at a private clinic or by giving the sample directly to the woman. It's important to be very clear on your role in the child's life and to know legally where you stand, so it would be worth getting independent legal advice before donating. The HFEA regulates all UK clinics, so you can be sure that treatment will be safe and according to the law. You won't have any legal rights or responsibilities for any children born as a result of your donation.

You can also provide a sample at a private clinic for use by someone you don't know. In the UK, sperm donors can donate sperm for up to 10 families and be paid up to £35 per clinic visit.

Twenty years ago, when I was at university, I remember some male friends discussing how donating at the local sperm bank might be a good earner. None of them ever went. They probably realised the money – while an all right sum for a student – wasn't worth potentially being contacted in the future by a mini-me if the law changed. Since then, it *has* changed – donors are only anonymous if they donated before 2005 (although the donor can now choose to have that anonymity removed). *See* page 144 for details. According to figures obtained by *The Times*, after the law changed the number of women treated with donated sperm fell by nearly a fifth in one year – 2727 in 2005 to 2107 in 2006.

## EGG DONATION

You can donate eggs to family members, but there are some restrictions, as with sperm donation.

You can also donate eggs at a private clinic for use by someone you don't know. You won't have any legal rights or responsibilities for any children born as a result of your donation. Usually you need to be between 18 and 36 years of age to donate, and some clinics will require your body mass index (BMI) to be within a certain range. And you will have to undergo various tests to make sure you don't pass on any medical conditions to the baby or mother.

Donating eggs is much more involved than donating sperm. You have to be a pretty altruistic person to go through the process – taking drugs to boost your egg supply, undergoing general anaesthetic during egg collection, being prepared for someone to contact you later in life. The whole process takes about three to four weeks. Egg donors get up to £750 per cycle of donation.

## WHAT TYPE OF PERSON DONATES?

According to the latest HFEA stats, over the last decade there has been an increase in the proportion of both sperm donors and egg donors (not egg sharers – *see* page 149) who don't have their own children. Around 70 per cent of sperm donors and egg donors were white British, while the second largest ethnic group was 'any other white background', highlighting the social and cultural barriers that clinics face in recruiting people to donate and the issues you may face to find a donor if you're from a black, Asian or minority ethnic (BAME) background.

Wendy Martin, Fertility Therapist at the Bristol Centre for Reproductive Medicine (BCRM), says…

'In my experience, there are three types of egg donors: women who voluntarily offer to donate their eggs to strangers out of the goodness of their heart, women who donate eggs to a blood relative, and "egg sharers" who donate in order to get lower cost treatment themselves.

'I've learned over time that there are characteristics that typify donors – they are empathetic and generous; they are also happy to go through the IVF process; they see their eggs as "cells" and not as a potential baby of their own and are happy to have contact with any donor-conceived adults that are interested in finding out about their genetic origins. It is also clear that prospective donors really "get" how hard it is for those who are struggling to conceive a child. They somehow know and understand that this is an extremely painful thing to go through and they genuinely want to do something to help. Donors feel lucky to have had the children they have and will say, "If I was in that situation and I knew that egg donation was the only way I could have children, then I would hope someone would do the same for me", a kind of reciprocal empathy. Sometimes donors who have young children will say, "I can't imagine what it would be like if I could never have had my children" and this is the incentive for them to help others try and achieve a family.

'In my experience, none of the egg donors I see believe that any baby conceived is "their child". They are very clear that they are not "the mother" of any baby that might be born as a result of their donation. They know, beyond a shadow of a doubt, that the woman who bears the child, who gives birth to it, and who brings it up, is the child's mother. Conversely, the women who see any child born from their egg as "their child" never donate their eggs. Even though it is just one cell, they would see it as "giving their baby away" and so just cannot contemplate the idea of doing such an impossible thing.

'Donor women (and their partners if they have one), appear to be completely comfortable and relaxed with being contacted by a donor-conceived adult. They say things like: "Well, if they want to come and see me, to see what I look like, or ask me any questions about their genetic heritage, their medical history, or why they might be the way they are, then I'll be very happy to oblige." They don't necessarily have any sense of what, if any, relationship might come from that initial contact, but they are open to seeing how things unfold.

'The fact is, donors have to possess every one of these characteristics and if they fall down on any of them it is unlikely they will come forward to offer their eggs. For example, if they don't feel they have sufficient time and can't fit it all into their hectic and demanding life; or if they don't feel the £750 they are given towards their expenses would be a sufficient incentive for them to make that much effort; or if they are not happy to meet any future adults conceived from their eggs; or if they are terrified of needles – or any other of the many reasons why they couldn't face doing it – they simply don't come forward. That is why egg donors are so rare and special and are such sought-after human beings.'

## EGG SHARING

Egg sharing is when someone going through IVF donates eggs collected during their treatment. It is seen as somewhat controversial, though, because the treatment is often offered to patients at a drastically reduced fee if they agree for any spare eggs to be donated. Of course, this is to try to increase egg donations, as numbers are low. But ethics committees have debated long and hard as to whether to agree to this – and, indeed, some clinics don't offer egg sharing.

HFEA stats show that, in 2013, 533 patients registered as egg sharers – a drop from 2012, when there were 629, and 2011, when there were 708.

## GOING SOLO

While men also have a ticking biological clock, women tend to run out of time earlier. With all the opportunities that now exist for women, we're often busy progressing our careers, travelling the world, exploring new ventures, and don't necessarily meet 'The One' in our most fertile years of our teens and 20s – if ever.

### Olivia's solo journey

Olivia was 32 when she met her last boyfriend. During their four years together, they decided they would have kids. But then they split up.

'At that stage I was 36. I'm not the type of person to go from boyfriend to boyfriend. But I wanted a baby. I didn't want to go on a date and sit in front of someone and go, "Hello, nice to meet you, will you be the father of my child?" Also, I'd been really burnt by the last relationship. I knew it would be a while before I met someone else – and I was scared. So I thought, right, I'm going to do this on my own.

'The biggest thing for me was the ethics of having a baby on my own. I remember going on a walk with work friends, and the subject of having a baby on your own came up, without me mentioning it. And the friend said, "It's really selfish, isn't it" – probably because she thought having one parent only would put a child at a disadvantage.

'I started looking into it all, joining the Donor Conception Network (DCN), who have different groups for all sorts of different parents – solo mums, gay couples, and so on. I went to a conference where I met donor-conceived children, some who were in their late 20s, who talked about their experiences in a positive way. I also remember ►

meeting one heterosexual couple, where they had used the husband's brother's sperm – and so they called him the "sp-uncle"!

'I also read Susan Golombok's book, *Modern Families*, which looks at all sorts of family set-ups, including solo mums. As solo mums have to self-fund, her research showed that they tend to be older and well-educated with disposable incomes, providing a very stable home. For example, my son has never been around any conflict. I once shouted at my mum and he looked surprised, because he wasn't used to anyone shouting. So there are little advantages like that. Golombok's research really helped me to frame in my mind what I thought the reality was for these children.'

Olivia went through IVF with a Danish clinic – buying the drugs at Asda where 'they do cut-price IVF drugs!' [although this isn't recommended by fertility clinics], having scans at King's College Hospital in London, before flying out to Denmark to have her eggs out and later the embryo transfer.

'I initially decided to do IVF with a Danish clinic as it was cheaper. I paid roughly the equivalent of £5000, and the deal was roughly three cycles for the price of one. I started by trying IUI, but the chances aren't great with it and – at about £500 a pop – it's quite an expensive way of doing it. So after four goes, the clinic said just do IVF. And it worked first time. But I also loved the clinic – it felt like no big bother to them – they would say "yes, we can do that", and they never tried to sell anything extra.

'I didn't go through IVF because of fertility issues, and so I didn't go into it with a sense of anxiety that some people would. It was a good experience for me.'

Olivia sourced the sperm from the European Sperm Bank, where you can choose an open or an anonymous donor. She chose open, so that when her son is 18, he can track down the donor if he wants to. The donor isn't obliged to meet him, though.

The European Sperm Bank had a greater range of donors on offer than the clinic where she had the treatment. After paying a fee, she was able to search their website and filter her preferences, such as height, weight, eye and hair colour. For an extra fee she could access the donor's full medical records, family background and get a photo of them when they were young. ▶

'I was looking for someone who was tall (as most of my family are tall), and dark haired with blue/green eyes as we all have eyes like that. I actually know quite a lot about him – he's American, his mum was a single mum with a law degree, his grandmother was a Taiwanese war bride and his grandfather is of German heritage. There was also a letter from him – so he writes a general letter to anyone who uses his sperm – and also a pen portrait [of him as an adult] by the nurses, and a photo from when he was about three. I can see a lot of similarities in my son in the photo I've got of the donor. But everyone says my son also looks like me.

'I spent a lot of evenings looking through the website. People say it's like online dating, because it is, which is slightly weird. Just like online dating, you get drawn into it. But when I did find the donor it felt like a click – he was head and shoulders above anyone else.

'I would love to meet him. And that's the one thing I hope I've got right. I hope my son doesn't feel in any way some loss or psychological distress that he doesn't know who this person is. The advice from the Donor Conception Network (DCN) is that you talk about it completely openly, before they can even speak. Back in the day, parents were told never to say anything – so lots of children grew up not knowing. There are now lots of books out there to normalise it.'

Olivia is not alone. There are plenty of people going solo. According to HFEA figures, of all women accessing fertility treatment (fresh IVF and donor insemination) with donated gametes in 2013, 17 per cent had no registered partner.

(*Name has been changed for privacy.)

## EMBRYO DONATION

You can donate embryos for use in treatment or research. You can't donate anonymously (*see* page 144 for details), but you won't have any legal rights or responsibilities for any children born as a result of your donation. Usually you need to be between 18 and 36 years of age to donate an egg and 18 to 41 to donate sperm, and you will have to undergo various tests to make sure that you don't pass on any medical conditions to the baby or mother. If your embryos were created using donated eggs or sperm, the donor will have to have consented to any subsequent embryo being used in this way, and donor sperm cannot be used for more than 10 families.

## Giving consent

When filling in our consent forms, Max and I had different views on the questions about how any spare embryos could be used. I happily ticked every box agreeing to the use of any spares for training purposes. Max and I took along our consent forms to the next consultation meeting with one of the nurses. She read through the documents and then pointed out that Max had not consented to any embryos being used for training purposes. Rather than face a discussion in public on the ethics of whether an embryo was already a life at just a few days old, I backed down and amended my form.

Max and I have been so incredibly lucky to have our children, and I recognise that only through scientific research and training has the procedure of IVF been honed over the years to the success rates seen today. So I wanted others to have this chance. And if that meant trainee embryologists using our spare embryos then I was happy with that. Max was not. But I respected his views. He is a practising Catholic, whereas I'm an atheist. Religion aside, it was an interesting moment on our IVF journey.

You may well experience a similar situation if you have a partner. To avoid any embarrassment or awkwardness when you meet the nurse or consultant, I would suggest discussing your views with your partner in private when you're completing the consent forms.

# Where to get help

## Egg banks
Some examples of egg banks:
www.londoneggbank.com
www.city-fertility.com/egg-donation-in-the-uk
https://crgh.co.uk/european-egg-bank/

## Sperm, Egg and Embryo Donation (SEED) Trust
This charity is a good source of information on donation.
https://seedtrust.org.uk

## Donor Conception Network
This is a good support network for people considering using a donor, or for families with donor-conceived children. The website has lots of advice and useful sources.
www.dcnetwork.org

## Q&A

**Nina Barnsley, Director of the Donor Conception Network (DCN)**

**Q. What services and support does the DCN offer?**
**A.** The DCN is a support network for anyone considering using donor conception [DC], as well as for families once they have children created this way. We focus on openness and building confidence and do this mainly through peer-to-peer support. We run local meet-ups around the UK and Ireland for people to connect, and we run two national conferences each year when people at all stages can get together. We also have a helpline and spend a lot of time helping people think through their hopes, anxieties, doubts and dreams. The website has a wealth of information and personal stories as well as a forum for members. We also run workshops for people considering

donor conception. We publish and sell a wide range of books to support parents in being open with their children and the wider community, and we also have a range of books for children to help them understand their origins. We also run 'Telling and Talking' workshops where parents can explore how to be open with their children.

There can be a lot of anxiety around the impact on the child, understandably, and many prospective parents are curious about the long-term outcomes for DC families. Our charity has been around for over 25 years, which provides us with a long view of family life, and in our network we now have donor-conceived adults having children of their own. Our decades of experience make us a leader in this field.

**Q. What advice would you give to patients considering using a donor?**

**A.** As with most things in life, the more preparation you can do the better. Explore your options, speak to us at the DCN and people who already have children. Try to remember that this baby will grow into a child and then an adult who may have questions (and opinions!) about their origins. Give them a story you are proud of.

**Q. Does your advice vary according to the patient situation?**

**A.** Our advice is very similar for all family situations, with some small differences. For single people we often encourage them to think about their resources and support systems – family, friends and community – and start building that network as soon as possible. Treatment can be gruelling and raising a child is a tough, expensive job, even for two people. For single people and same-sex couples it's worth being prepared for questions that may come much sooner than for heterosexual couples, as it will be obvious that they must have had help of some kind to create a baby. The questions can come from children asking about why their family is different, or wondering about their dad (or mum for gay couples). Questions from other adults will mostly come from genuine interest and curiosity, but it is worth preparing for what to say to overly nosy people who you don't necessarily want to share all the most intimate elements of a child's beginnings with.

**Q. What is the biggest decision or challenge for patients considering using a donor?**

**A.** Using a donor is a different way to have a family. Having and raising a child who is genetically connected to people outside the family is different to conceiving a child with a couple's own eggs and sperm. Raising a child who is not genetically connected to you is also different. Deciding where to have treatment and choosing a donor can be difficult. Couples may not both be in agreement about using donor conception and it can take time and effort to resolve that. Parents, depending on their circumstances, often feel a deep grief that they couldn't use their own eggs or sperm, or their partner's eggs or sperm, or that they don't have a partner to share this with.

It's worth being aware that children can also feel a sense of loss at not being genetically connected to a side of the family they feel very attached to or can feel sad being cut off from their donor and his or her wider family. Donor-conceived people may feel a lot of curiosity about their donor and other genetic family and that can sometimes feel threatening to parents, or can be difficult if there is no information available for a child. Some children in solo or same-sex families may miss not having a dad or a mum. This is not to say that they are unhappy with their parent(s) or their family as they can be separate feelings.

As with most parenting, being open, honest, warm and caring, as well as listening deeply and not being too reactive if issues come up, will support families through the majority of life's challenges. Being part of a support network like the DCN can also be invaluable.

**Q. Where would you recommend patients sourcing eggs/ sperm/embryos from?**
**A.** We don't recommend particular clinics. It is a very personal and often complex decision. We would recommend that people invest time in the decision, as it is such an important one, and ideally speak to others who have chosen a variety of different options to see which route feels right.

## CHAPTER 5

# **Cryopreservation**

## Freezing eggs, sperm and embryos

alf a century ago, freezing life would have sounded like science fiction. But these days, egg, sperm and embryo freezing is fairly commonplace with regard to fertility treatment. In 2018, 38 per cent of all IVF cycles involved frozen embryos. And storage cycles have shot up by 523 per cent, rising from 1,500 cycles in 2013 to almost 9,000 in 2018. Meanwhile, the use of fresh embryos has dropped – down 11 per cent between 2013–2018.

There are all sorts of reasons why you might want to freeze embryos: if the treatment doesn't work; you want to try for a sibling; you want to take a break from treatment or you need to stop treatment halfway through, for example if you over-respond to drugs or develop a medical condition; you're going through a life change that might result in being unable to try for children in the future (such as the risk of being injured if you're in the police or armed forces, or you're planning to go through gender reassignment surgery).

Jheni's story…

From our first cycle of IVF, Max and I didn't have any other embryos that were high enough quality to freeze. But our second cycle produced two high-quality embryos, so one was transferred immediately (but that round didn't work), while the other was ▶

frozen. We ended up using this frozen embryo six months later and it developed into our second daughter. We always joke that she is a very chilled character, and maybe that comes from having been 'put on ice' for a while.

I've got friends whose kids are sort of like twins – the embryos both fertilised together, one was immediately transferred to the mum's uterus and was born later that year, while the other was frozen and then defrosted a year and a half later.

Other friends or patients I've chatted to have actually decided in advance to freeze all their embryos after fertilisation, rather than transfer a 'fresh' embryo straight away. More on that later... First, let's find out about the process of freezing – or so-called cryopreservation.

## HOW FREEZING WORKS

To freeze an embryo, it is placed in a special solution containing 'cryoprotectants', and then cooled, before being stored in liquid nitrogen at about -196 degrees C.

Essentially, the cryoprotectants act like a sort of antifreeze. They are vital to protect the cell against the damage that would be caused by ice crystals if they were able to form inside the cell. It would be a bit like if you filled a glass bottle to the brim with water and put it in the freezer – it would eventually explode because the ice would increase the volume and break the glass of the bottle. Some of the cryoprotectants are large sugar molecules that can't pass through the membrane of the embryo. Maybe you remember your biology lesson on osmosis, where water passes through a semi-permeable membrane from an area of higher concentration to an area of lower concentration? Well, as the concentration of cryoprotectant sugar molecules is higher outside the embryo, water molecules are drawn out through its membrane in order to balance out the difference in concentration.

At the same time, cryoprotectants contain other smaller molecules, such as ethylene glycol or glycerol, that can pass through the membrane. This is to ensure that the embryo doesn't become too dehydrated and shrivel up like a raisin, causing irrevocable damage.

A new fast-freezing technique called 'vitrification' is growing in popularity. Vitrification literally means 'transforming a substance into glass'. It differs from the traditional slow-freezing cryopreservation in that it uses three to four times higher concentrations of cryoprotectants, and cools the embryos 10,000 times faster by plunging them directly into liquid nitrogen.

When the time is right, embryos are defrosted essentially by reversing the process – warming the embryo very carefully in air and a water bath, and gradually diluting the cryoprotectants, so that as the cells rehydrate, they don't blow up. Embryos are then left to rest before being implanted two to four hours after reaching body temperature.

Embryos can be frozen when they are at different stages of their development – when they're just a single cell, right up to when they are a multicellular blastocyst. Now, you may have heard of places that are freezing whole human bodies in liquid nitrogen in the hope that one day they'll be able to bring them back to life (the cartoon *Futurama* went a step further and just froze heads in the belief that technology will advance enough to grow organs and limbs). In reality, whole human bodies – or heads – are so complex and contain so many cells that defrosting them in the future will be an almost impossible challenge. But embryos have relatively low numbers of cells and are incredibly small – a blastocyst is only about a tenth of a millimetre in size. Hence, cryopreserving and then defrosting them is much easier.

Many clinics will only freeze embryos that meet certain criteria, as poor-quality embryos don't survive the freezing process well and are less likely to result in a pregnancy. For example, if an embryo has a lot of 'fragmentation' (whereby too many fragments mean the cells are not dividing correctly), then the chance of it successfully defrosting is lower than for a higher grade embryo.

## Dr Cesar Diaz-Garcia, Medical Director IVI London, says…

'During vitrification, the temperature of the embryo decreases at a rate [that would be equivalent] of around 10,000 degrees a minute, which means that we can get to almost below -196 degrees C in milliseconds. This avoids ice crystal formation.'

## Paul Wilson, BCRM Head of Embryology and Andrology, says…

'Ice crystal formation and cryoprotectant toxicity are the enemies when freezing embryos. Ice crystal formation may lead to cell membrane damage, thereby reducing cell and embryo survival rates, and cryoprotectant toxicity may reduce the implantation potential of the cells that do survive. With the older "slow-freezing" techniques, the water in the embryo cells is gradually removed and replaced using cryoprotectant solutions, the whole process taking about 2.5 to 3 hours from start to finish. This extended period of exposure allows a long time for ice crystals to form and for the embryos to be exposed to the risks of toxicity. With vitrification, higher concentrations of cryoprotectants, used for much shorter periods of time alongside very rapid cooling rates, mean the embryo goes from being in a liquid state to being "vitrified" in a fraction of a ▷

second, which doesn't allow ice crystals of any significant size to form or, potentially, to form at all.

'When we thaw the embryo, we want it to come through the warming process looking exactly as it did the moment we vitrified it. These days, in the vast majority of cases, the embryos come out looking the same as they did when frozen and their implantation potential appears to be comparable to embryos which have not been frozen.'

When a frozen embryo is transferred depends on your personal situation. If you have regular periods, the clinic may simply thaw out and transfer the embryo within your natural cycle, and a series of scans can confirm when your endometrium is at the optimum thickness ready for implantation. But if you have irregular periods, your consultant may recommend using drugs to control the process by suppressing your natural cycle and triggering a fake period, and then taking more drugs to boost the endometrium lining. (*See* page 68).

## COSTS

Thawing and transferring an embryo to the uterus costs on average anywhere between £800 and £1500, while storing an embryo costs between £170 and £400 a year. A number of high-quality embryos can be stored together – and often the cost of freezing is the same for one embryo as for several. In NHS-funded cycles, storage fees are covered for one year.

Although an embryo won't necessarily survive the freezing and thawing process, the length of time that a frozen embryo is stored doesn't affect the chances of getting pregnant.

Usually, clinics will store embryos for 10 years, but in special circumstances embryos can be stored for up to 55 years. It's important to tell a clinic if you ever change your contact details, as after the specified time period they are entitled to discard stored embryos if they can't get hold of you.

## SUCCESS RATES

Birth rates for treatment cycles using frozen embryos are now comparable with those using 'fresh' embryos transferred straight after fertilisation. In 2017, success rates for frozen cycles were slightly higher at 23 per cent, compared to 21 per cent for fresh cycles. When figures were broken down into age bands, under 35s had slightly higher success rates with fresh cycles, but over 35s were higher with frozen embryos. It's worth bearing in mind that this could have been because results were skewed by embryos being frozen when patients were younger and more fertile.

Dr Chandra says…

'Previously, successful defrosting only resulted in a pregnancy rate of about 25 per cent or so. Whereas now, when you freeze blastocysts, on average the thaw rate is around 90–95 per cent. And, once you have defrosted it, then success rates following frozen blastocysts are virtually equivalent to fresh. So, nowadays freezing is considered as no big deal.'

Dr Cesar says…

'If you have the perfect hormonal conditions and you are young enough, it doesn't matter if you transfer a fresh or a frozen embryo. But freezing embryos without a justification (risk of OHSS, hormonal imbalances, logistic reasons…) is not scientifically supported.'

'Freezing embryos can be a way of avoiding patients having ovarian hyperstimulation syndrome (OHSS) [*see* page 71]. So, for example, for a patient at risk of developing OHSS, you can wait to see if the risk is high before considering doing a fresh rather than a frozen embryo transfer.'

## ELECTIVE FREEZING

There is currently a trend for so-called elective freezing – deciding in advance to freeze all embryos and intentionally delay embryo transfer for a few weeks or months, rather than transferring an embryo immediately after fertilisation in a fresh cycle. This could be for a number of reasons. Sometimes patients want to build in a break from the process to give themselves a bit of breathing space. There is also some evidence that having a break lets the woman's body readjust and rid itself of all the egg-boosting and egg-releasing drugs. And other research suggests that babies born from frozen embryos are closer in birth weight to those conceived naturally, as babies from fresh cycle IVF have been known to have a lower birth weight, which can affect health later on.

In the US, around a quarter of IVF cycles now use the 'freeze-all embryos' strategy. However, the HFEA have given 'elective freezing' an amber light rating (*see* page 118). This is because experts aren't sure yet whether freeze-all cycles really are more effective. Some recent research suggested no benefit. Published in 2019, the study of 460 women at clinics in Denmark, Sweden and Spain showed a tiny difference in success rates – 26 per cent for freeze-all cycles versus 29 per cent for one embryo transferred on a fresh cycle. But a large-scale clinical trial called E-Freeze is due to release results soon, which should hopefully help to clarify the debate.

> Paul Wilson says…
>
> 'There's a school of thought out there – and some interesting data – that suggests the stimulation of the ovaries may disrupt the endometrium in some way. By separating out the two events (create the embryos in the stimulation phase, freeze them, and then put them back when the endometrium has not been exposed to the stimulation drugs), a more receptive endometrium may result, and higher success rates be obtained.'

## CONSENT

Before freezing embryos, there will be all sorts of consent forms to sign. For example, you can agree for any unused embryos to be used for research or training. And you will need to specify your wishes should your circumstances change, such as in the case of a divorce or death. At any time before an embryo is transferred or used for research or training, a partner (or a donor) can withdraw consent.

## EGG FREEZING

In the US, companies like Apple and Facebook are now offering egg freezing as a perk to lure in potential female employees. Some companies based in the UK, such as Goldman Sachs, are following suit. The idea is to preserve fertility by freezing eggs at a younger age (when eggs are of a higher quality), so women can focus on their careers and establish financial security in their 20s and 30s, and not panic that they've yet to meet 'The One' or they're not ready to become a solo parent. As we know, the stats show that with each year that passes the chances of a woman conceiving get slimmer, because the quality and number of eggs drops (*see* page 18).

While some question the ethics of encouraging women to delay having children during their natural childbearing years and see these 'job perks' as more of a bribe, personally I wish that I'd been more aware of the age at which fertility starts to decline and had the option to freeze eggs. However, 20 years ago when I was in my early 20s, the technology was not as advanced as it is now, and any frozen eggs may not have survived the process in any case. But techniques are now so advanced and thawing rates so successful that for the next generation this is a truly viable option. Indeed, if it's appropriate, I may well encourage my girls when they are older to consider 'social freezing' (as it's known in the industry).

Of course, there are all sorts of other reasons you may want to freeze your eggs. Just like with freezing embryos, you may have a medical condition, be about to undergo surgery or have a high-risk job. Your consultant will be able to talk you through options.

And, if you are considering a donor egg, it is worth knowing that there are now egg banks that store donated frozen eggs (*see* page 179).

Dr Chandra says...

'With fresh egg donation, you've got to synchronise the period between the donor and the recipient. So both have to start treatment at the same time, because the recipient has to be ready for the embryo transfer at the same time as the donor. Previously, supply and demand was such that patients used to have to wait for six months or a year for fresh donated eggs. Now, with advances in vitrification, success rates with frozen donor eggs are as good as that with fresh donor eggs; hence you can access donor eggs on demand, at a time that suits you.'

## WHAT'S INVOLVED IN EGG FREEZING?

First, you'll need to have a test to check for infectious diseases, so that if you have any such disease your eggs can be stored separately from others to avoid any risk of contamination. Then you'll go down the usual IVF path and spend a few weeks taking drugs to boost your egg supply and ensure they mature, ready for collection (*see* page 73). But after the eggs are extracted, instead of being fertilised in the normal way during IVF, the eggs will be cryopreserved, either by the traditional slow-freezing method or by the faster process of vitrification (*see* page 160). The clinic will probably aim to freeze around 15 eggs, which are then stored in liquid nitrogen.

You will have to give written consent for an amount of time you wish to store the eggs – usually 10 years, but up to 55 years in special circumstances. It's really important to let the clinic know any changes to contact details, so they can get in touch with you when the consent period is up, otherwise they'll have to discard the eggs.

You'll also need to fill in forms clarifying how your eggs can be used, such as for research or training, or what will happen to them in the event of your death.

Finally, when you're ready to use the eggs, they will be thawed and fertilised using the ICSI method, where the sperm is injected into the egg (*see* page 89), as freezing can make the outer membrane tougher than normal.

Paul Wilson says…

'Historically, and until very recently, we have preferred to freeze embryos rather than eggs – frozen eggs had variable thaw survival rates, reduced fertilisation, embryo development and implantation rates compared to non-frozen eggs, and so we had more confidence with embryo freezing than egg freezing. (This was particularly important when considering fertility preservation cases where we might have only had one chance ▶

of preserving a woman's fertility.) The reason for the poorer outcomes observed was likely to be because the egg cell is one single very large cell [as opposed to a multi-cellular embryo with many smaller cells]. Cryoprotectants need to penetrate across the whole width of a cell to be effective and it's technically harder to achieve this with increasing cell size and, therefore, you're more likely to get variable survival rates with eggs than with embryos. Also, we just didn't know the best way to freeze eggs with our knowledge at the time. Everything improved dramatically with the introduction of vitrification. The evidence now published shows very high survival rates for most patient groups and fertilisation/development/implantation rates largely comparable to non-frozen eggs.'

## SUCCESS RATES

Egg freezing is the fastest growing fertility treatment type. According to the HFEA's latest trends report, egg freezing increased by 240 per cent from 2013 to 2018. Yet stats show that in 2017, in the UK, only 19 per cent of IVF treatments using a patient's own frozen eggs were successful. So it's worth keeping success rates in mind when considering whether to freeze your eggs, as doing so does not guarantee a baby in the future. The HFEA and Royal College of Obstetricians and Gynaecologists (RCOG) are encouraging clinics to be more open with patients about the relatively low success rates, so that they can make informed decisions.

Some research has suggested that using frozen eggs leads to higher rates of miscarriage, but the sample sizes of the studies were limited as relatively few IVF babies have been born from the patient's own frozen eggs.

## WHEN SHOULD YOU FREEZE YOUR EGGS?

Everyone's fertility varies. A lucky few get pregnant naturally in their 40s, while others (like myself) start to lose their fertility at a much younger age. But it's worth bearing in mind that our eggs are of higher quality when we're younger and hence more fertile. So experts at the Royal College of Obstetricians and Gynaecologists say that the best time to freeze eggs is in your early 20s. But obviously don't panic if you're well past this age, as plenty of people get pregnant from eggs frozen when they're older. Indeed, research shows that if a woman freezes her eggs before she turns 35, the chances of success are higher than conceiving naturally as she gets older.

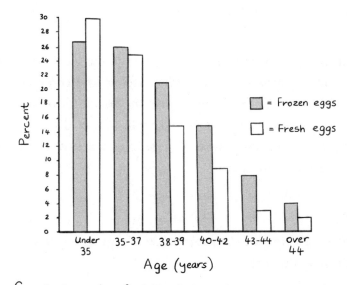

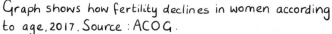

Graph shows how fertility declines in women according to age, 2017. Source: ACOG.

Barbara Scott MARR, MAR, MFHT, Chair of the
Association of Reproductive Reflexologists, Author,
Lecturer, says…

'What is being taught in schools [about fertility] is in the main incredibly poor. We are quite rightly teaching our young people how *not* to get pregnant. However, we also need to teach them that their fertility is finite. There is now a huge campaign to try and ensure that people are aware of this. So many women are already over 35 and don't realise that their fertility is likely to be impaired. Men are included in this too; males over the age of 40 are likely to see a significant drop in the quality of their sperm. We need to ensure that all of our young people are given the information to allow them to make informed choices.'

Interestingly, a study in the US that was published in 2016 asked reproductive experts whether fertility decline and cryopreservation should be discussed when patients visit the doctor for routine check-ups. Most experts felt that doctors should initiate discussion about fertility decline, but not bring up egg freezing, unless it was in relation to other medical treatment.

## COSTS

Expect to pay up to £8000 for the whole process. Here's a rough breakdown of the costs:

- £3350 – egg collection and freezing
- £500–£1500 – drugs
- £125–£350/year – storage
- £2500 – egg thawing and transfer to uterus

It's worth knowing that if you've got a medical condition that needs treatment that is likely to affect your fertility, such as going through chemotherapy, you may be able to receive funding.

'I had my eggs frozen in 2015. I was 39 at the time. A long-term relationship had just finished. I wanted to have children and knew that, statistically, by the time I met the right person and felt ready to commit to that person by having children together, the quality of my eggs would have deteriorated.

'In France, this procedure is illegal.* So my French gyne [doctor] advised me of three clinics she could recommend, in Belgium, Spain and Cyprus. The procedure involved being on site for a week. It was winter time. So I chose Cyprus! The medical side cost about 1500 euros in total. Then add flights and hotel.

'When the time came to use my eggs, I was very busy with work. So I had the eggs transported to the UK – the whole process took about three weeks, cost about £1500 and a fair amount of paperwork, but it was easy to go through. Once there, the eggs were fertilised and then one was implanted.' ANNE

## OVARIAN TISSUE FREEZING

If you're unable to freeze your eggs or embryos, some clinics offer ovarian tissue freezing. This involves extracting either a whole ovary, or bits of tissue from an ovary that contains eggs, freezing and storing them until you are ready to have them transplanted back into your

*In France, egg freezing is currently only allowed in cases where a patient is likely to become infertile after medical treatments (such as chemotherapy), or for egg donors. But this may change soon, as new bioethics laws have been proposed.

body. It could be an option if you're about to go through chemotherapy and there isn't time to collect your eggs, or for prepubescent girls whose eggs aren't mature enough but they need medical treatment that may affect their fertility. It's early days for the technique, which does carry risks, such as the possibility of reintroducing cancerous cells back into the body. It's worth discussing this option in depth with consultants and other professionals treating you for medical conditions.

### Info for transgender people

If you're about to go through gender reassignment treatment, you may not be thinking about your future fertility. As hormone therapy can impact on fertility, it might be worth you considering freezing eggs or sperm in case you would like to have a family in the future.

## SPERM FREEZING

Before sperm is frozen, its quality is assessed against all the usual factors, such as concentration and motility (*see* page 41), and checked for infectious diseases so that, if necessary, it can be stored separately to avoid contamination. The sperm is then mixed with a solution of cryoprotectants, and divided into a number of different containers (known as 'straws'), before being cooled and stored in liquid nitrogen.

Roughly half of the sperm will become damaged through the freezing process, but each sample produces so many that this isn't a problem. The good news is that IVF using frozen sperm is just as successful as IVF using fresh sperm.

You'll need to fill out various consent forms to confirm how long you want your sperm stored for, what should happen to it in the event of your death, and whether any leftover sperm can be donated or used in research and training. You can change your mind about any of these decisions before treatment or before sperm is used in research or training.

When you're ready, you can defrost a batch for use in exactly the same way as fresh sperm is in IVF, ICSI or IUI. Any other batches of sperm can remain in storage for later use.

Recent research suggests that long-term sperm freezing makes little difference to live birth rates. As with eggs and embryos, sperm samples are usually only stored for a maximum of 10 years, but in some special cases sperm can be stashed away for up to 55 years. If the man is going through treatment or needs an operation, then sometimes the NHS funds storage. But the average cost of freezing sperm is between £175 and £450 a year.

## WHY FREEZE SPERM?

Freezing your sperm could be useful if you have a low sperm count, poor sperm quality, or you struggle to produce a sample after your partner's eggs have been extracted (let's face it, it's a lot of pressure to perform in that brief window of time). But freezing your sperm could also be a good option if there's a risk of injury through your job, such as if you're in the police or armed forces. Or maybe you've got a medical condition and will need to go through treatment, such as chemotherapy, which could result in subsequent infertility. You might also want to consider it if you're planning to go through gender reassignment, or in case you want children in the future and do not want to risk a reverse vasectomy failing.

## TESTICULAR TISSUE FREEZING

This involves freezing a small piece of tissue from a testicle and then storing it either as individual cells or as one piece of tissue. While the technique is still in the research phase, the idea would be to either inject or transplant cells or tissue back into the body at a later date, or possibly produce sperm from these cells in a lab. This could be an option for men who are unable to produce sperm or to preserve fertility for prepubescent boys undergoing cancer treatment.

## LEGAL ISSUES

There is an ongoing discussion over the length of time that women are allowed to store their frozen eggs. Currently, most women are only allowed to store their eggs for 10 years (or up to 55 years in special circumstances, such as if a woman might become infertile through chemotherapy). There have been calls to extend this time period, as many feel it doesn't reflect the capability of IVF today. Indeed, in 2019, a group of women brought the UK's first legal challenge to the 10-year limit on preserving frozen eggs. The HFEA have said this is a matter for parliament to change legislation.

The complexity of different cases also means it can be hard to find the right moral ground. In Australia in 2016, there was a case where a dead man's testes were removed and put into storage in case his partner wanted to use his sperm in the future for IVF, because sperm must be retrieved and stored within 36 hours of death in order to be useable, and ideally within 24 hours. But his parents have contested this as the couple had only been dating for seven months. The same year, the French authorities allowed a woman to take the sperm her husband froze before he died to Spain for IVF, as it's not legal to carry out post-mortem insemination in France. This is legal in the UK.

CASE STUDY

**Having a dead husband's baby**

Isabelle and David* met when they were at sixth-form college, got married and decided to try for children. But after some time trying, they resorted to IVF – undergoing treatment in the country where they were living at the time. Fertility treatment can be a lot cheaper abroad, but success rates vary (*see* page 128). After a number of cycles of IVF, the couple still hadn't managed to conceive. And Isabelle had a terrible IVF experience in one particular country that almost put her off altogether – she doesn't go into details, simply describing it as 'traumatic'.

When they eventually returned to the UK, they decided to try IVF again. Just as they were starting the consultation process, David woke up one morning seeing a strange 'floater' in his eye. So he went to the optician to get it checked out. The optician spotted some swelling behind the eye and sent him to the hospital to have that looked at.

It transpired that he had a large brain tumour. Within two weeks, he was undergoing biopsy surgery. That same day, Isabelle picked up the IVF drugs to start treatment.

'The doctors asked me: "Are you sure you want to go through IVF right now?" I said that we'd been trying to conceive for years, so "yes",' says Isabelle. 'And it felt at the time that, while everything else was going wrong, this was our "good thing". But in hindsight it was potentially silly. I was taking the IVF drugs while David was having brain surgery.'

The IVF cycle didn't work. They tried again, this time at Guy's Hospital, because it has a special unit where they treat cancer patients undergoing chemotherapy – and provide counselling. It didn't work either. They tried again. This time Isabelle got pregnant, but then suffered an ectopic pregnancy – where the embryo attaches outside the uterus. By this time, David was undergoing chemotherapy every month.

'Our bedroom was like a pharmacy,' says Isabelle. 'David questioned whether we should be going through IVF again. I said: "Don't you want us to?" And he said: "I didn't mean that." It all got really emotional and stressed, on top of his treatment.

'What I've realised since is that he didn't have the capacity to support me, and I didn't really realise what I needed, and therefore didn't really support him in the right way. For a while we were off on our own little "fix-it" missions. I felt like "Let's get pregnant and everything will be fine", he felt "Let's get rid of my brain tumour and everything will be fine". And for a time that's how we coped. And really, we did great. We did really well to get through, and we could communicate in a way I've seen few couples be able to since. We had to be so very vulnerable and honest with each other, and we shared total absolute highs and lows. I've tried not to look back and question decisions we made, because at the time they felt right and they're done now and can't be changed, but I'm not sure it was helpful to our situation to be doing IVF. But at the time it gave me something positive to focus on, so maybe it did help. Either way, it was tough.'

Two weeks after Isabelle recovered from the ectopic pregnancy. David suffered a seizure, and suddenly went from basically healthy and without symptoms, even though 'undergoing treatment', to being critically ill.

'This was the first time doctors started using the word "dying",' says Isabelle.

Two months later, David died.

'When I told my parents I wanted to try again for a baby, they were mostly worried that I wouldn't be able to handle it if I tried IVF, or more specifically ICSI, and it didn't work. The people I told outside of our sphere thought it must be a knee-jerk reaction to losing David as they didn't know we'd even tried before.'

Just before David's chemotherapy treatment, the oncologist had talked with him and Isabelle about freezing his sperm, as they were of child-bearing age and it's often suggested in that case, whether the cancer sufferer is male or female. The NHS offers this for free, as the effects of chemotherapy on fertility are unknown and vary between patients.

After David had the seizure, Isabelle realised he wasn't going to get better. She got in touch with Diane Blood, whose case changed UK law ▶

about using a dead partner's sperm. Diane's husband, Stephen, caught meningitis in February 1995, two months after trying to start a family. His rapid decline into a coma meant he never signed consent forms agreeing that his sperm could be used. The 1990 Human Fertilisation and Embryology Act banned Diane from using Stephen's sperm without his written consent – the Human Fertilisation and Embryology (Deceased Fathers) Act was passed in 2003, allowing sperm taken from a male now deceased to be used to fertilise an egg, as long as the man and woman were married (or living together as man and wife) or had been receiving treatment together at a licensed IVF clinic. But in 1997, a court ruled that Diane could use Stephen's sperm to try to conceive a child. She now has two sons, who are 19 and 15. Both were conceived through IVF, using sperm harvested when Stephen was in a coma, just days before he died.

'I wrote to Diane, explaining my situation, and she advised us to write letters to each other and to our doctor saying we would like to have children together and were trying to do that despite the cancer and chemotherapy,' says Isabelle. 'Very emotionally we wrote those together and they went on both our doctors' files.'

Isabelle herself is now contacted from time to time by other widows with frozen eggs, sperm and/or embryos, to ask about her experience as they make their own decisions.

After David's death in December, Isabelle openly admits she had a breakdown.

'It had been so incredibly intense for a year, especially the last few months, then when David was gone there was just emptiness and nothing to do but be consumed by grief. I was a total mess. I had five months off work. I went to Thailand for a month. For some of that time I drank a lot, for some of it I stopped eating. I wasn't sleeping well – and was on sleeping tablets every night. Everything had happened so quickly. But one focus I had was to write down our whole story. I relived David's last few months, which helped me understand what had happened. It was incredibly therapeutic – along with yoga and cycling. But at some point, around when I went back to work two days a week, I had a real sense of "you've got to turn this around", especially if I was to try for a baby.'

▶

Isabelle sought help from naturopath, nutritionist and fertility coach Kathleen Boyd, who runs Birds & Bees in Putney. Kathleen advised her to do a six-week detox.

'I committed 100 per cent and quickly I felt amazing in comparison to the previous few months. I never went back to work full time. I did acupuncture, yoga, meditation, lots of cycling, lots of walking outdoors. So lots of "me care". By that time I decided I was ready to try again. The hospital demanded a letter from my counsellor stating she thought I was emotionally strong enough to try, which they'd insisted on from the start and which my counsellor was happy to provide.

'So fourteen months after David died, Mum came with me to the six-week scan. The nurse remembered David and cried. I remember hearing the heartbeat going "ba boom, ba boom" and cried.'

Isabelle now has a wonderfully active, happy little two-year-old. She's clambering on the sofa, as I chat to Isabelle in her cosy home. The sitting room is filled with photos of her and David, from adventures in exotic-looking lands to wedding photos to childhood photos, slightly frayed by time.

Her daughter certainly looks very like her father from the photos – particularly her eyes.

'At the beginning she really looked like him. Now, she'll pull an expression which is just like David – and she's never even met him. She's like a real-life nature/nurture experiment.

'Previously, I wouldn't have shared with people that I was going through IVF. But now, once I explain that my husband died a number of years ago, people realise it must have been IVF. It's quite refreshing, as people get fixated on the other side of the story, as opposed to the IVF side. It's sad that people feel they can't talk about it openly whatever reason they're having it.'

(*Names have been changed for privacy)

# Where to get help

## HFEA Choose a clinic
The HFEA's useful 'Choose a clinic' service, where you enter a postcode and hone your search options, such as finding clinics that use donor recruitment.
www.hfea.gov.uk/choose-a-clinic/clinic-search

## Donor Conception Network
This is a good support network for families of donor-conceived children. But they also have lots of resources for patients with different situations.
www.dcnetwork.org

## Egg banks
There are a few clinics around the country that store frozen donated eggs, so donor and recipient cycles don't need to be synchronised. Some examples:
www.londoneggbank.com
www.city-fertility.com/egg-donation-in-the-uk
https://crgh.co.uk/european-egg-bank/

# CHAPTER 6

# When IVF doesn't work

## How to cope and prepare for the next step

This is the chapter you probably don't want to read, but if you haven't been successful with IVF, or you've decided it's time to draw a line and accept that IVF isn't going to work for you, then hopefully this chapter will help.

The average live birth rate for each embryo transferred for women of any age is 23 per cent. This means that for most people, IVF is unlikely to work first time round – and in many cases it may never work. Understandably, this can be absolutely devastating.

The ex-chair of the HFEA, Lisa Jardine, once described to the BBC how the IVF world is a 'market in hope'. The media – and often clinics – tend to focus on successes and not the reality that IVF won't work in, on average, 77 per cent of cases. No one talks about the grief and sense of failure experienced by many, time and time again.

In order to understand what it must feel like to go through many failed cycles, I have spoken to experts and to people who have experienced this, and to those for whom IVF has never worked. Through their words, I hope to help those in similar situations.

'After the first cycle of IVF we had a miscarriage. That's when it hit me what was ahead and I thought maybe it's not going to work. We took a break, as I couldn't face going straight back into it. The second time round [using a frozen embryo from the first cycle] I had emotional help and was in a much better place, feeling quite positive and calm. But it didn't work. So when we did another fresh cycle, I wasn't expecting it to work either. This time, the miscarriage happened early on. By this point I'd been through so much that it didn't knock me as much. I think you do get a bit resilient to it.' **ALANA**

'Each time it didn't work, I felt really gutted that all the emotion, time and energy had been totally wasted, but mainly worried that it might never be possible to conceive, which just felt really sad.' **SOPHIE**

## A NEGATIVE RESULT

After so much emotional and financial investment, when you first see a negative result on the pregnancy testing kit it can be really hard to process. You might feel angry that you've been through so much or that no one at the clinic seems to be able to tell you why it hasn't worked. You may look around for someone or something to blame. But most of all you will probably feel like a failure. It's really normal to have these feelings. Go easy on yourself. IVF isn't for the faint-hearted and anyone who has been through the whole process knows the heavy toll it takes.

'I feel that IVF was sold to us as "Do this and you'll have your baby. This will be the miracle cure. Although they never said you will get pregnant, they said it might happen."' **ALANA**

Initially, nothing is likely to make you feel better. You will probably need some time to grieve for what could have been. With time, the shock and devastation does ease. While you may feel like rushing back into doing another cycle of treatment straight away, it's probably best to give yourself a bit of time to recover physically and, maybe more importantly, mentally.

Harder still may be if the pregnancy test shows a positive result, but then in the following weeks you get your period. Miscarriages are actually quite common for everyone, regardless of whether you've been through IVF or not. So the clinic is still unlikely to be able to tell you why you've had a miscarriage.

If you do suffer a miscarriage following IVF treatment, it may be a small comfort to learn that researchers at the University of Aberdeen, who studied more than 100,000 women, found that the chance of getting pregnant from future treatment was 10 per cent higher for women who had previously had a miscarriage than for those who had not become pregnant at all.

Not all miscarriages result in bleeding, though. In some cases, the foetus dies but the uterus doesn't empty of blood, so the woman may not realise she's lost the baby. This can be a devastating shock if you believe that you're pregnant and then at the first scan no heartbeat is detected.

Another difficult scenario is having an ectopic pregnancy, which is when the embryo implants outside the uterus. This can still happen if you go through IVF because, although the embryo is placed into the uterus, occasionally it can move and implant in other places – in the case of an ectopic pregnancy, this is usually in the fallopian tubes. Contact your clinic if you're experiencing pain in your abdomen and bleeding that looks unusual – watery and dark brown in colour. It's important to treat an ectopic pregnancy early to avoid damage to the tubes. If a tube ruptures, you may experience sharp, intense pain in your abdomen, and feel dizzy or sick. You'll need to get emergency treatment immediately.

## DEALING WITH INSENSITIVE PEOPLE

We've all been there – confronted by a situation where someone seems to find getting pregnant as easy as blowing their nose. Most of my friends for whom this is the case have been incredibly sensitive, particularly after finding out we were struggling to conceive. But, of course, there are colleagues, associates and strangers who have no knowledge of what's going on in your private life. And some may even give you a wry smile and joke: 'Come on. Get on with it. The clock is ticking.' You smile back through gritted teeth. Yes, thank you for that. Very helpful.

When you're desperate to have a baby, insensitive people are everywhere.

> 'You have to be prepared. Some people who you would expect or want more from will not react in the way you want them to. They will say the wrong things. And some people, who you might have hardly any relationship with at all, will say the most profound and beautiful things.' **JESSICA**

### Jheni's story...

The way I coped with anyone asking the tricky question about whether we have kids or are planning to have them was to just volunteer the information up front and be very open about saying that we were going through IVF. But, of course, you might not be able or want to do this with everyone and so you need to be prepped for insensitive comments and tricky situations.

Just before we started the first round of IVF, I remember someone coming into the office where I was working at the time with a cake – to celebrate her becoming pregnant. A cake! Firstly, I thought to myself, who does that sort of thing?! Don't people just show the baby's scan to their nearest and dearest? Secondly, in this enlightened day and age where the media often feature couples struggling to conceive, surely you're aware of the fact that other people around you may be trying for kids – unsuccessfully.

Before this, I'd managed to stay positive about everything – even when every time I walked anywhere it seemed like I passed yet another pregnant woman. But I didn't know this lady, and felt nothing for her, except for a pang of... was that jealousy? It floored me. I remember having to take myself away from the situation, seeking refuge in the toilets to just have a moment out. All I could think was: 'I really really hope IVF works for us.'

Another time, I remember just after our failed cycle, one of the mums at my swim group told us she was pregnant and then said she hadn't timed it well and wished she was due in March and not July, as it would fit better with when she'd like to take maternity leave. As I already had a child, she probably didn't think anything of telling me this. But it still felt like a kick in the stomach after the failed cycle that I'd just been through.

Coping with insensitive people can be really tough. After my own experiences, I've always tried to be incredibly sensitive to the situation of others – I've found that it's always better to assume someone is struggling to conceive than risk offending them.

When researching this book, I attended a fertility conference when I was fairly pregnant. Despite it being an unusually hot winter's day, I tried to keep my bulging stomach as inconspicuous as possible under baggy layers and a carefully positioned scarf. Sweating profusely throughout the day, I think I managed to pull it off, as no one seemed to be aware I was pregnant.

I also tried to hide the pregnancy from a colleague at work, who I knew had been through numerous failed cycles of IVF. Eventually, when I could hide my protruding tummy no longer, she came up to congratulate me. She was lovely. I told her that I'd been dreading her finding out. She was so positive about it and simply said that it actually helped her in a way as it gave her hope that IVF might work for her one day.

The reality is that, for many of us, going through IVF is a gruelling marathon, where often there is no finish line in sight, and it can end up bringing out the worst in us.

## THE GREEN-EYED MONSTER

'Women often tell me that they think they're going mad – or are bad,' says Wendy Martin, Fertility Therapist at the Bristol Centre for Reproductive Medicine (BCRM). 'They get feelings of being completely out of control of their emotions, finding themselves full of rage, hatred and extreme jealousy, being utterly obsessed and preoccupied with thoughts about babies and other women's pregnancies. We are socialised to be "nice" and "pleasant" – even in our thoughts. We know it is not good to be jealous and hate-filled, especially if it is to do with something as wonderful and benign as the announcement of a pregnancy or the birth of a baby. I reassure patients that this is completely normal and they aren't bad people.

'I remember once this lady I was counselling through IVF told me that her sister-in-law had four children and she was planning her fifth. The sister-in-law had worked it out that if she got pregnant that month, the baby would probably be born on St Nicholas' Day, and if so then she would call it Nicholas. What an insensitive thing to say to someone who is trying with IVF! And the lady later told me that was exactly what happened!'

To cope with moments like these it's probably best to prepare for them, so that they don't floor you when someone makes an insensitive comment or you come up against a challenging situation in public. Maybe sit down and have a think about how open you want to be about going through IVF. What will you say to people when they ask if you have kids – or if you would like to have them? How will you navigate yourself away from an upsetting scenario?

What coping mechanisms do you have in place to stay positive after a tricky situation? How will you react when someone tells you their bit of good news?

And, crucially, take the pressure off by not putting yourself in situations that are going to cause you pain.

Jheni's story…

Before going through IVF the first time, a friend was organising another friend's baby shower in London. I had been on the road with work on and off for a number of months and was pretty exhausted physically. So I felt I didn't have the emotional strength to be all upbeat at the friend's baby shower. I made my excuses that I was still going to be abroad at the time.

My friends were really great at being understanding. Many admitted later that they were nervous of telling me that they were pregnant when they knew we were going through IVF.

'Family and friends were pretty good about it all. We would make the effort to go and see them and their kids. But they completely understood that when it came to birthday parties we didn't want to go – it would be too much to cope with when there would be, say, 10 couples there, all with their kids. When parents are all together, they talk a lot more about being parents than when it's just us and another couple with their child.' **PIP**

'I expected that other people would be more mindful of what we were going through. Slowly I came to realise I couldn't expect that other people know how I'm feeling and behave accordingly. So instead I had to plan for things like when someone taps you at work and says, "Guess what? We're pregnant!"' **RICHARD**

'The thing I struggle with most is pregnancies. I find that harder than seeing children. I made the mistake once of going out with my three friends with all their kids. I felt like I was missing something. I now don't put myself in that situation. I just see them one-to-one. My friends understand. What I've learnt over the years is that you have to protect yourself.' ALANA

## SEEKING SUPPORT

Many people I've spoken to say that online chat forums have really helped them. Speaking to other people, from all around the world, who have had similar experiences normalises our own behaviour and feelings. It helps us to realise that we're not the only ones dealing with this. Others have said that keeping a journal or writing a blog has been therapeutic or helped them to reach out to others.

'It took me a long time to acknowledge to myself that I was really struggling at times and there was a lot of self-loathing, because it was male factor infertility. And it took me a long time to talk to someone. The one thing I learnt was that you must talk – find a confidante.' RICHARD

While talking to supportive family and friends is also a great way to navigate through the challenges of IVF, sometimes it can be really useful to speak to a professional counsellor. They will be experienced in giving advice specifically on fertility issues. They also won't know your family history or have any other agenda. They will be able to help you to see things in a different light, away from the pressure of close relationships.

'Often people have heard IVF treatment is an "emotional roller coaster". So they think that the treatment itself is difficult and become afraid of how the drugs are going to affect them emotionally and physically – they assume the treatment is the "roller coaster", says fertility therapist Wendy Martin. 'If a couple get pregnant the first time of doing IVF, and they walk away from the experience knowing that they are going to have a baby, they might be forgiven for thinking, "It wasn't that bad, was it? The injections weren't nice, and I had a few symptoms, but it wasn't as awful as we had both feared."

'What is really difficult is when IVF fails – or worse still, when it works and a positive pregnancy is achieved but at the six- or twelve-week scan the pregnancy is found to be non-viable and a miscarriage ensues. The profound and powerful grief that is experienced when treatment doesn't work can come as a great shock to the couple. And the differences in how the couple each deal with the grief can also add to the stress as they may not understand why each other are responding so differently.

'The difficulty is compounded if, after a number of different treatments, the longed-for baby still eludes them. This is the real roller coaster, and nobody can prepare themselves for it. The cycle of hope and despair associated with repeated failures of assisted conception treatment is probably one of the most challenging emotional and psychological experiences any individual or couple will ever go through. The abject fear of never having a family can be overwhelming. This is when support is really needed.

'Most people benefit from taking some time to think about what helps them cope in their lives, what activities or attitudes help them get through when they face life's challenges. I also teach simple mindfulness techniques and make bespoke self-hypnosis recordings (on their phones) to help them with sleep problems and any anxieties and insecurities.'

'I knew how much stress it placed on us, my wife in particular with having to deal with work and all the hormones, and going through the process again was not something to look forward to.' **ED**

'You feel like your body is a slave to IVF. If the last round of IVF hadn't worked for us, we weren't going to do it again. It's no life to live for such an extended period of time, with no way of knowing if it will ever work. Each time IVF failed, we dealt with it by thinking if we weren't going to be able to have kids, then we had to make our lives worth living. We went on holiday to Belize. We immersed ourselves in the things that we love doing – going to Devon, paddle-boarding, kayaking and walking. It helped, but we were on the verge of giving up and not trying again, drastically changing our lives to go and live abroad.' **PIP**

'When it didn't work I felt very disappointed, because it felt like knowing what the problem was would fix it, but it brought a new load of doubts.' **NICKY**

## Trying for a second child

If you've already had a child through IVF, you may just feel incredibly lucky and not want any more children or not want to go through the process again. But some people may want to try to have another child. Some friends I know have actually got pregnant naturally after having their first child through IVF. Others, like ourselves, have tried again with IVF and been successful. Others had a child that was conceived naturally, but then hadn't been able to get pregnant again, suffering numerous miscarriages before considering trying with IVF. ▶

If you're like us and you experienced a failed cycle second time round, then you'll know how devastating that can feel. I remember the exact moment when I realised the cycle had failed. It's the moment that every hopeful-mother-to-be dreads – the red specks. It sounds ridiculous, but I wasn't prepared to have a period. I was two days off taking the pregnancy test that would signal whether our second cycle of IVF treatment had worked. As it worked first time on our first cycle of IVF and we have a wonderful daughter, I was probably a bit too overconfident that it would work again.

I'd read that sometimes pregnant women bleed slightly. But over the course of the day, the orangey-red specks developed into a heavier flow of deeper mahogany. There was no escaping the fact that these were no mere specks of blood, but the womb lining leaving my body.

I'm working in an office. The day started out well, writing about an interesting scientific voyage to the depths of the ocean, enjoying banter with my colleagues, making cups of tea and chatting to friends round the water cooler. But after the trip to the toilet, this rapidly turns into clock-watching. And all I want to do is leave.

I just want to go and buy a pregnancy test and confirm my worst suspicions. But first and foremost, I want to see my little girl. To hold her close. I can smell her already. Panic sets in – what if something has happened to her too? No, don't be illogical, you know she's safe and well. Our lovely childminder would have called if something was wrong. She's fine.

Thoughts swirl in my head – swinging from optimism to self-pity to blame to optimism again. Maybe, just maybe, I am pregnant. I surreptitiously check the NHS website on my phone for info on bleeding during pregnancy. Some women apparently bleed slightly all through pregnancy. But this isn't slight.

By the time I actually get round to doing the pregnancy test, I am so exhausted from a day wracked with emotion that I have no energy left to care. That evening we are supposed to have friends pop round for a drink for a belated celebration of Max's birthday. We cancel. All I want to do is curl up on the sofa and watch guilty-pleasure TV, forget and escape.

The next morning I wake up to that weird feeling when you know something is wrong, but you can't remember what. It's like the morning you're due to take an exam, but you haven't yet remembered that you have to – and then reality kicks in and you get that sinking feeling in your stomach.

Now, I wish I hadn't told so many people that we were trying again. It means every time I see a friend I have to say again that it hasn't worked this time, listen to their condolences, say we have an embryo in the freezer and hopefully it will work next time.

But will it? That is the big question on my mind. I know we have no money left – we've actually had to borrow from the bank to make the final IVF payment. It will be quite a while before we can afford to try again – and my biological clock is ticking.

And that's the crux of it. How many cycles of IVF can we afford? How much money should we throw at trying to have another baby instead of spending that money on experiences for our current family of three? When should we discuss how many times we're prepared to go through this? And how many times should I put my body through ingesting all those drugs?

The irony is that before we started trying again with IVF, I didn't want another child. My little girl satisfied every part of me. I didn't want another baby interfering with our special relationship, taking me away from time with her. (And maybe I was scared that IVF wouldn't work again and the whole lengthy process would be harrowing and in vain.) But then I thought about how special my relationship is with my sister. How much we need each other, love each other, rely on each other.

Our consultant, Dr Chandra, suggested it would be worth trying sooner rather than later – at that stage we had no idea whether my fertility was declining rapidly, and the stats (*see* page 19) for getting pregnant get lower and lower year on year. I was 39 and counting. Knowing the stats can mess with your mind.

▶

Once we decided to try for another child, I really started wanting one. It's not just like saying to your partner, how about we start trying again and then you keep an eye on the ovulation sticks for the optimum timing. This involves numerous visits to the clinic for consultations, blood tests, sperm samples. It involves a team of at least 10 people knowing you're trying. It involves pumping yourself with drugs, giving your body up to the hands of science. It involves going under general anaesthetic and having your eggs sucked out of you. It involves your partner masturbating on cue in a small room next door. It involves lying spreadeagled on your back while a friendly nurse inserts an embryo. It involves friends and family subtly asking the time frame of when you might know if it worked.

Maybe arrogantly, I thought that as it worked first time for us last time, it would work first time again. I ensured everything we did was exactly the same. I didn't drink a drop in the build-up or through the process, I stopped exercising to fatten up and get my BMI at the right level, my reflexologist came to treat me again on a regular basis. But what I hadn't factored in was that our life was different now.

We had a little girl to look after. She was still only eight months old. That's a full-time job in itself. I was back at work in an office two days a week, and writing this book in any 'downtime' when the little one was asleep. Add into the mix that we'd just started a loft conversion (with plans to put a lodger up there to help us get through the next few years of childcare payments before free schooling kicked in). And so life was certainly busier than before.

In retrospect, we had taken on too much. I was exhausted by everything. Who knows whether my body just couldn't cope – or whether the high-grade embryo that was put back in just wasn't actually up to scratch. But that fateful bleed happened straight after a hectic day of shouting down the phone at the bathroom store lady about another undelivered item, while swearing at the server, which had decided to go on strike on deadline day for the magazine I was working on.

Inevitably, I blamed myself for failing to get pregnant this time round.

'If it doesn't work, a lot of women believe it's definitely their fault,' says fertility specialist Wendy Martin. 'Even if the partner has low fertility, the woman still thinks that she's to blame, as the sperm fertilised the egg, and the embryos all grew nicely in the lab, but the moment they were put back into her womb, it didn't work. So she believes she did something wrong.'

Logical me still partly blamed myself. But I also had a niggling thought in the back of my mind that it was a bit Max's fault too. I found myself forgetting that during all the treatment, he'd cooked every evening, fed our little girl the last bottle before bed every night, spoilt me with foot massages; despite being stupidly busy at work he had made it home for bath time almost every evening. Instead I remembered when he hadn't got up in the night to get our little one back to sleep, how he'd been out with friends on his birthday to watch a film (that I hadn't wanted to see anyway, so we hadn't got in a babysitter)...

In retrospect, I didn't handle the situation well. If you've been through something similar, you may well feel the same. One of the best bits of advice I got from a friend (who had been through IVF herself) was be kind to yourself – and give yourself a break, you're only human.

## MOVING ON

Very sadly, for some people IVF never works. Deciding when to stop having treatments is an incredibly difficult decision.

Lesley Pyne is the author of *Finding Joy Beyond Childlessness*. She went through six failed rounds of IVF and then, at the age of 40, decided to call it a day. Many dark years followed, although she now says she loves her life. But to get to this point was a long, challenging journey of recovery.

'We decided to stop trying when I was 40 as the chances of success drop significantly around that age. It was easier to stick with our decision because we'd had enough by then. I think even if someone had given us another free go, we'd probably have said no. We were done physically and emotionally.'

Understandably, for Lesley it wasn't an easy road to her current happy, confident state. She got through the tough times by first learning Neuro-Linguistic Programming (NLP), 'which helped me to understand what was going on in my head, and so started my healing process', and then later by a mixture of yoga and traditional therapy.

'I've come out the other side as a different person. A friend of mine was saying to me the other day, I look lighter. Well, I've lost a bit of weight, but it's not that. For the first time in my life I feel comfortable in my own skin. I paint my nails and wear leopard-skin boots, and things like that, but that's an outward sign of being confident enough and comfortable in who I am. I was never like that before.'

Over the years, Lesley has met others who haven't been able to have children. 'More to Life' is a community run by Fertility Network UK for men and women who are childless not by choice. The community has helped them to deal with the sadness and to build an inner strength to deal with questions such as 'Do you have children?'

'We were really fortunate to meet a group of about 15 of us who have stayed long-term friends. Some of these are my closest friends, because we understand each other like nobody else.'

Over time, Lesley has found that for her and her husband there are some benefits to not having children. 'There's a flexibility. Both my husband and myself have the freedom to explore who we are, and do different hobbies and travel. Perhaps we couldn't have done these things if we'd had children.'

So Lesley's main message is that the future can be bright. 'It makes me really sad when people come out of this and think I'm always going to be sad. That's absolutely not true. There is a grieving process to go through, but there can be a happy ending. You can find joy at the end of it.'

Lesley is just one of many who have gone through a challenging journey of accepting childlessness and come out the other side. Author Jessica Hepburn went through 11 failed cycles of IVF, but at the age of 43 decided to draw the line under it.

When I interviewed her, she explained how it was incredibly therapeutic to write about her experience in her first book, *The Pursuit of Motherhood*.

'The moment I "came out" and was not secretive about this experience, it made it so much easier. I just wasn't carrying it in the same heavy way. The act of talking about it is helpful.'

Jessica has since become a pioneer on raising awareness about struggling to conceive. She founded Fertility Fest – an arts festival focused on infertility and modern families.

'It's become a social mission for me. There's been the perfect storm of legalising abortion, the pill and IVF, which has facilitated reproductive choice, enabling women to focus on careers and be more than wives and mothers. But because fertility declines much earlier in women than men and IVF isn't a perfect science, it has also created a very complex situation as well. What I advocate is that there are many routes to parenthood and we just need more information earlier on… before people are in a position of pain and desperation. So that they can make rational decisions and the best decisions, not only for themselves, but for the children they're bringing into the world.'

Jessica feels that women entering the bamboozling world of fertility options may not be given the best advice for them at the right stage. Older women need to be given the hard stats about how age affects fertility and, hence, be guided by clinics towards the best option for them for their age.

Just like Lesley, Jessica says she has found happiness despite not having a child. In the book, she describes how she is 'living the fullest life imaginable without children' and adds 'I recognise that the life I am having is not the one I wanted, but it's a pretty special one and as life is so short we've got to make the most of every second we're given on this planet.'

If IVF isn't working for you, make sure you keep communicating with the clinic about what else you can try and the potential steps you can take going forward.

One of the toughest things will be deciding when to stop trying with IVF. Discuss this with your partner (if you have one). After a failed cycle, it's easy to get drawn into trying 'just one more time' and not wanting to give up as the next cycle could be the one where it works. Your consultant will be able to advise from a medical perspective on the chances that further cycles will be successful. But it's important to consider whether you can afford it, the potential strain on your relationship, and also how you yourself are coping physically and mentally. Only you know how far you are prepared to go to try to have a child.

One of the key messages I learnt from talking to patients for whom IVF hasn't worked is that it's OK to stop if you feel it might be the right time to do so. Inevitably, you are likely to feel very sad about ending your IVF journey, but maybe also you'll feel a huge sense of relief. All these stories, and my own IVF saga, go to show what an involved process fertility treatment is, both physically and emotionally. Whether going through it as a couple or on your own, it is one of the most challenging – if not the most challenging – thing you'll ever do in life. Life can be harsh – it can knock you down and it can scar you. But hopefully we all find ways to cope and continue to enjoy it – whether with or without children.

## SURROGACY AND ADOPTION

If IVF hasn't worked for you, you might want to consider other options, such as surrogacy or adoption.

Surrogacy is when another woman carries and gives birth to your baby. 'Full surrogacy' involves your eggs or those of a donor being used. 'Partial surrogacy' involves the surrogate's egg being fertilised with your partner's sperm. Surrogates usually receive around £10,000–£15,000. You'll need to factor in clinic costs as well – depending on your circumstances, this may just be the cost of IUI. It's important to know that, in the UK, the surrogate is the legal mother until you get a parental order from the court, so make sure that you consult a lawyer before going down this route.

**Surrogacy organisations:**

Surrogacy UK – surrogacyuk.org

Brilliant Beginnings – www.brilliantbeginnings.co.uk

Childlessness Overcome Through Surrogacy (COTS) – www.surrogacy.org.uk

Adoption is when a child who can't be brought up within their birth family becomes a full, permanent and legal member of a new family. As with surrogacy, adoption is legally complicated and so it is worth consulting a lawyer.

**Adoption support:**

Adoption UK forum – allows prospective adopters and adoptive parents to share knowledge and support each other – www.adoptionuk.org/forums

First4adoption – the national adoption information service for England – www.first4adoption.org.uk/adoption-support/

'We're nearing the end of our IVF journey, as I am feeling quite tired of it. I can't keep doing it for much longer. Next year will be three years of trying with IVF. It takes over your life. It's a massive weight. I can't actually remember what it feels like when I didn't have this. I might have a lovely time on holiday or whatever, but it's always there. One little trigger can bring it back. We still desperately want our own family. But I try to think I'm lucky to have my husband. I'm lucky to have so many things in life.' **ALANA**

'At that time, I felt like having a baby should be a natural organic process. I took it for granted that everyone can have children. Having gone through the whole experience of having fertility problems to going through treatment to having a family has taught me humility and compassion and not to take things for granted. I now realise that life goes on with or without children.' **CHAMPA**

# Where to get help

### Your clinic
All clinics licensed by the HFEA have to offer you counselling before you start treatment. Some clinics will offer it for free, while others may require payment.

### More to Life
Fertility Network UK organise events for people who are childless not by choice.
https://fertilitynetworkuk.org/events/mtlmeetup/

### Gateway Women
Website and online community for women united by and beyond childlessness.
https://gateway-women.com

### British Infertility Counselling Association
A directory of accredited private therapists, some of whom also provide telephone and video counselling.
www.bica.net

### British Association of Counselling and Psychotherapy
www.bacp.co.uk

## CHAPTER 7

# What's next for IVF?

The recent big breakthroughs and the future of fertility treatments – artificial embryos, gene editing, designer babies

J ust over 40 years ago, the birth of Louise Brown, the first IVF baby, raised concerns about 'Frankenbabies' and 'playing God'. Yet today, more than six million babies have been born this way, and in many countries all around the world it is an accepted and celebrated medical treatment.

In that time, IVF has come on in leaps and bounds, honed by professionals intent on creating families. But as with any medical procedure, regulators have had to keep tight control of its development, particularly as it involves creating life. And regulation varies between countries. For example, in the UK there has been an increase in the use of IVF in female same-sex couples, while the technique is only legal for heterosexual couples in some other countries. Embryo freezing is legal in many countries around the world, but not in Italy. And although, in the US, pre-implantation genetic diagnosis (PGD) during IVF can be used to select an embryo's sex for 'family balancing' (*see* pages 129 and 215), in the UK it can only be used by patients with a family history of a serious genetic condition to avoid it being passed on to their children.

Of course, scientists are always pushing the boundaries and the goalposts are constantly changing, so ethics committees are working hard to keep up with the developing science.

## CURRENT BIG TRENDS IN THE UK

Stats taken from HFEA data taken in 2017/2018 and published in 2019/2020.

### TREATMENT TYPE

**93%** of patients undergoing fertility treatment are having IVF (2017)

There was a 3% decrease in ICSI (where the sperm is injected directly in the egg) between 2016 and 2017, maybe because clinics now feel it's necessary in fewer cases.

### EGG OR SPERM DONATION

**13%** of IVF cycles used donated eggs or sperm (up 3% between 2012 and 2017)

Egg sharing has been declining since 2011

### PATIENT SITUATION UNDERGOING IVF

Heterosexual couple: 90.7% (2017), 94.4% (2018)

Female same-sex partnership: 5.9% (2017), 3.1% (2018)

No partner: 3% (2017), 2% (2018)

Surrogate: 0.4% (2017), 0.5% (2018)

## AVERAGE PATIENT AGE

**35.5** years for IVF (65% are under 37) (2017)

**34.5** years for donor insemination (73% are under 37) (2017)

## AVERAGE SUCCESS RATES

**23%** IVF birth rate (per embryo transferred) but **31% for women under 35** (2018)

**14%** Donor insemination birth rate (per treatment cycle) (2017)

## PERCENTAGE OF FERTILITY TREATMENT FUNDED BY NHS

**60%** Scotland (up from 42% in 2012)

**45%** Northern Ireland (down from 48% in 2012)

**41%** Wales (up from 28% in 2012)

**35%** England (down from 39% in 2012)

## MULTIPLE BIRTH RATES

**8%** in 2018 (down from 24% in 2008)

## EMBRYO FREEZING

In 2018, 38% of all IVF cycles used frozen embryos, compared to using fresh embryos, which decreased by 11% between 2013 and 2018. This increase could be down to clinics wanting to reduce the number of embryos transferred at one time to reduce multiple births.

**23% birth rate per frozen embryo,** compared to **21% for cycles using fresh embryos (2017)**

## EGG FREEZING

**240% increase** in egg freezing between 2013 and 2018. This increase could be due to people wanting to delay childbearing and more awareness of fertility preservation, particularly for patients with cancer or transgender patients.

Jessica Hepburn, author of *The Pursuit of Motherhood, 21 Miles* and founder of Fertility Fest, says…

'I campaign about improved fertility information for young people, because if people really understood what this technology can do and can't do, then it would be a much more emancipating technology than it is. I knew of one woman who was told to freeze her eggs at 42! And the worst thing I hear is that a woman on her own who is in her early 40s makes the decision to go for sperm donation. It's been a massive process for her to think about solo motherhood and going for sperm donation. What she hasn't thought about at all is that she might need egg donation. I always say, "Please, save some money." There's just not enough public understanding about better success rates with different ways of making babies. Women need to be supported to make a decision early enough.'

## RECENT BREAKTHROUGHS

The following developments have just made the move out of the research lab and into fertility clinics, but it's still early days for the techniques…

## 'THREE-PARENT' BABIES

In April 2019, a baby boy was born in Greece using the genetic material of three people – the father, the mother and a donor. The experimental technique used sperm from the father, an egg from the mother and another egg from the donor.

The event caused huge controversy. The technique – known as 'mitochondrial replacement IVF' – is only supposed to be used in cases where a mother risks passing on a rare mitochondrial disease to their baby.

In the recent Greek case, however, the mother had no such genetic condition, and the procedure was carried out simply to help an infertile couple who had already been through four cycles of IVF.

Mitochondria are the 'power stations' of the cell, helping them to produce ATP – the molecular currency for transferring energy. Sperm only carry mitochondria in the tail. During fertilisation, the sperm head buries into the egg, leaving the tail outside. This is why mitochondrial diseases are only carried by the mother, as the sperm doesn't pass on any mitochondrial info to its offspring.

Mitochondrial diseases are relatively rare, but cruel. Roughly one in 200 children in the UK carries some form of genetic mutation that could result in a mitochondrial disease, which cause all sorts of illnesses affecting everything from the heart to the liver to the central nervous system. And babies born with these conditions may not even reach their first birthday.

In an attempt to thwart this cruel hand of fate, scientists developed mitochondrial replacement IVF. 'Mitochondrial transfer' or 'mitochondrial donation' involves one of two techniques. Maternal spindle transfer (MST) is when the DNA from a mother-to-be with faulty mitochondria is injected into a donor egg with healthy mitochondria, before being fertilised as normal by the partner's sperm under the usual IVF process. Pronuclear transfer (PNT) is when genetic material is transferred from an embryo created using the mother and partner's sperm into an embryo created using a donor egg. As the DNA of three different people are used, this has led to the technique being coined 'three-parent IVF' – although around 20,000 genes are from the actual mother compared to only 37 genes from the donor, just 0.1 per cent of the child's entire genome.

The US Food and Drug Administration (FDA) has yet to approve the technique. As mitochondria are also known to affect cell death and how fast nerves signal to one another, the FDA could be holding off because of concerns that not enough is known about long-term effects on health. But fears that this mitochondrial replacement IVF could lead to 'designer babies' are unfounded, as traits such as hair colour are controlled by DNA in the nucleus of a cell – and mitochondria sit outside the nucleus.

Following a decision in 2015 where Parliament voted to amend the 2008 Human Fertilisation and Embryology Act, UK clinics are now allowed to carry out mitochondrial replacement IVF for families that carry mitochondrial diseases. The UK is the first country to regulate mitochondrial donation. But only people with a very high risk of passing a serious mitochondrial disease on to their children are eligible for treatment.

If you have a mitochondrial disease, or think you may have one, then discuss this with your doctor, who will be able to refer you on. The HFEA needs to approve any mitochondrial donation.

## WOMB TRANSPLANTS

For female patients with infertility caused by problems with the uterus (such as if she was born without a womb or it was damaged during childbirth), it's now possible to have a uterus transplant – either from a living relative or from a deceased donor. The first baby to be born from a uterus transplant from a deceased donor was in 2017. The previous year, the uterus of a 45-year-old donor (who had died of a haemorrhage but had previously given birth three times) was transplanted into a 32-year-old woman, who had eight blastocysts frozen following IVF four months before. A number of babies have now been born this way.

## The personal touch

Mental health is high on the agenda at the moment and looks set to become more and more important in years to come. A huge part of going through the IVF process is dealing with the psychological side of it.

Start-ups are already specialising in concierge fertility services to take the stress out of the IVF process. Services include: dedicated fertility coaches on hand 24/7 to answer queries; personalised finance plans, sorting fertility bills into fixed monthly payments; IVF tourism, offering tailor-made trips abroad for cheaper treatment.

## THE NEXT STEP

According to experts, the following developments are just around the corner and may be coming to a fertility clinic near you in the next few years...

### NON-INVASIVE TESTING

Currently, embryologists can only find out information about an embryo and its genetic status by doing a biopsy. But when cells are removed, there is always a risk of the embryo being damaged. Another complication is that sometimes the cells that are analysed don't reflect the embryo as a whole.

Scientists are now researching whether it's possible to discover the necessary information about the embryo from the fluid that it sits in. The technique is still in its infancy, but there are already some promising results, with some suggesting that non-invasive testing of the fluid using 'cell-free DNA' could actually detect the embryo's genetic make-up better than the traditional biopsy method. It seems that in future it's highly likely that non-invasive testing will be used to assess embryos.

### Paul Wilson, BCRM Head of Embryology and Andrology, says…

'When you biopsy the embryo, you might happen to take a group of abnormal cells that have been pushed to the outside of the embryo, and so you could be labelling a healthy embryo an abnormal one. The Holy Grail would be to not have to do that invasive process at all, but to do non-invasive testing. This involves us looking at the droplet of culture fluid that the embryo has grown in to see if we can identify clues regarding viability, for example looking at embryonic DNA which has been shed by the embryo as it has developed in the laboratory. Work in this area is advancing rapidly, with some very encouraging data being published in the last couple of years. The approach taken is largely as per the existing prenatal cell-free DNA screening for conditions such as Down's syndrome, where there is testing for the foetal DNA shed into the mother's blood.'

### Dr Valentine says…

'A good analogy of non-invasive testing is to imagine you'd never met someone, but you went to have a look around their house. You would know what sort of person they are from their possessions – clothes, books, files… From all these fragments of their life, you can get an idea about their income, how many children they have. As an embryo develops, we now recognise they leave fragments of themselves that can tell you things.'

Dr Cesar Diaz-Garcia, Medical Director IVI London says...

'Non-invasive testing will become a reality very soon. There are already multiple trials assessing its performance. Although it is not a ready-to-use tool, it will be very soon – in the next couple of years...'

## VAGINAL MICROBIOME PROFILING

Inside and outside our bodies live all sorts of microorganisms – bacteria, fungi, viruses – that make up our 'microbiome'. In the last few years, we've heard more and more about how the microbes living inside our guts are indicative of our health. Well, the same seems to be true for the microbes in our vaginas, which research suggests play a key role in our reproductive health.

Studies have shown that the success of an embryo implanting in the endometrium is influenced by the presence of microbes. But it all depends on what type of microbes are there – some microbes seem to limit success, while others boost it. Various studies have found that live birth rate is lower when microbes such as *E. coli* (including both *Staphylococcus* and *Streptococcus* strains) are present, yet higher when *Lactobacillus* exists.

Microbiome research in relation to reproduction is still in its infancy. What we do know is that throughout a woman's life, hormonal and lifestyle changes affect the complex microbiome of the vagina, and more research is needed to understand how this impacts fertility. Maybe one day vaginal microbiome profiling will be one of the standard tests for patients going through IVF.

## ARTIFICIAL INTELLIGENCE

Considering the fertility industry is estimated to have generated $25bn (£19.10bn) to date, it's no wonder that large tech firms and small start-ups alike have been getting in on the act.

Already, there are a myriad of consumer apps, such as Flo and Mira, which can be downloaded to help couples trying to conceive naturally, providing info on things such as predicting ovulation and tracking hormone levels. But there is a new wave of companies and institutions turning their attention to how artificial intelligence (AI) might help patients trying to conceive.

Univfy is a Californian start-up that uses machine learning to crunch the data from patients' lab tests, such as age, BMI, fertility history and so on, to predict IVF success. Meanwhile, Canadian start-up Future Fertility has created the egg-scoring algorithm Violet, which they say can predict successful fertilisation with 90 per cent accuracy. It's currently less good at predicting things like embryo survival rate and implantation success, but the company says that will improve as the software is exposed to more and more data at IVF clinics from which it can 'learn'.

In 2019, researchers at Weill Cornell Medicine in the US used AI to help accurately identify whether embryos had a high chance of progressing to a successful pregnancy. The researchers trained an AI algorithm using a backlog of around 50,000 images of embryos of varying quality, and then used the software to assess patients' embryos to within about 97 per cent accuracy. The algorithm even outperformed embryologists.

Across the Pacific in Australia, a company called Life Whisperer has developed a similar AI tool that was trained using over 20,000 embryo images and had a 50 per cent better success rate than embryologists at predicting successful implantation. Various clinics around the world are currently testing out the software, and then the company will apply for regularity approval to take it to market.

At the moment, such AI-powered predictors are no guarantee of success. But it seems that one day machine learning could have a big role to play in fertility treatments.

## Dr Chandra says...

'Artificial intelligence is taking off in a big way – in the next 5–10 years, it will start being used more and more. AI is going to make sperm and embryo selection standardised and more consistent in the decision-making. Currently, the embryologist's decision is based on objective criteria, but inevitably there is some subjective bias and human error. In the future, it's not that we won't have embryologists – they will ultimately choose the embryos and do the decision-making – but AI algorithms will help. For example, the reason why many IVF cycles fail is that although the embryo may look great, it is chromosomally abnormal. The only way to know this is to do pre-implantation genetic screening (PGS). But many people can't afford it and it's invasive. If you used artificial intelligence, you would never know whether the chromosomal make-up is normal or not, but if the algorithm picks up an embryo which it knows that in, say, 100,000 people led to a pregnancy, then it helps to choose a "better looking" embryo for transplant. And AI will also help to tell people what their chances are of getting pregnant by using data from millions of patients who have been treated based on their age, hormone levels and everything. So AI will help to meet patient expectations, such as if a patient wants to know if they should aim for a family now or whether they can wait a few years.'

## IVF's influence on epigenetics

Epigenetics describes how lifestyle and the environment influences genes. The basic idea is that chemical tags, known as 'epigenetic marks', affect how genes are expressed (see page 141 for a description of the exact science of epigenetics).

But epigenetics is complicated, and scientists still don't know exactly how epigenetic marks are passed from one generation to the next. However, scientists are now considering how IVF might ▶

influence epigenetics. In other words, the IVF process might induce epigenetic changes to the blastocyst, which could then have health consequences (good or bad) for the resulting child.

Research on mice at the University of Southampton showed that, prior to implantation, the blastocyst is actively sensing its environment, and adapting its subsequent metabolism accordingly. If we apply this idea to IVF, it raises the question as to the influence on the developing embryo of the culture medium, which the embryo sits within in the Petri dish. Currently, scientists aren't sure what the ideal composition should be for the culture medium.

## THE FUTURE

While (most of) the following developments have yet to make it out of the research lab and into the mainstream, it may not be long before the techniques are being used by fertility clinics around the world...

### GENE EDITING

Gene editing is where DNA is inserted, deleted, modified or replaced in the genetic material of a living organism. In recent years, the gene editing technique known as 'CRISPR Cas-9' has been revolutionising the world of genetics, as it allows scientists to edit genes very precisely.

DNA is made up of sequences of so-called base pairs, which are combinations of four letters (A, C, G, T) that determine our characteristics. Using CRISPR, scientists can now target specific areas of a gene, correcting 'spelling mistakes' in the base pair letters and preventing genetic diseases. Over the last 10 years, scientists have used the technique to genetically modify various organisms, such as creating mosquitoes resistant to malaria and GM plants resistant to disease. Previously, any gene editing research in humans had not focused on eggs, sperm and embryos. But that is now changing.

In 2017, researchers in Portland, Oregon, managed to tweak gene variants associated with heart failure in a human embryo. However, they were only working on early stage embryos in the lab, which weren't allowed to develop for more than a few days.

But then in 2018, Chinese biophysicist He Jiankui dropped a bombshell. He claimed to have used CRISPR to make twin baby girls more resistant to HIV.

The HIV virus enters and infects cells by binding to a protein on the cell surface called CCR5. He claimed to have edited a CCR5 gene in a way that would cripple production of the protein, so that HIV would not recognise it.

Nicknamed Lulu and Nana, the twins were born in October 2018. He met with widespread criticism from scientists and others in the industry, who were concerned for the girls' well-being and outraged that he had flouted regulations that prohibit gene editing in human embryos if they are going to be used for reproduction.

Since then, it's been suggested that He's gene editing did not actually produce the desired result and could have caused unwanted or 'off-target' mutations. The Chinese authorities suspended He's research and began an enquiry into his work and the possible involvement of other scientists around the world. He has since gone missing.

In view of all this, there have been calls for a rapid review of the ethics and much tougher penalties for breaking the rules. However, in 2018, the Nuffield Council on Bioethics in the UK gave a cautious green light to embryo gene editing, provided it is in the best interests of the child, such as if the family has a history of a genetic disease. But the ethics body did highlight the importance of research into the safety of such gene editing, and discussion on the impact to society.

The key concern is that so little is known about side effects. While CRISPR is fantastic for targeting specific genes, there could be 'non-target' detrimental effects. In other words, one health problem would be fixed, but another health issue created.

So, while CRISPR looks very promising as a technique for targeting unwanted genes, it's got a long way to go until it will be deemed safe by the scientific establishment for human embryos used for reproduction.

## 'DESIGNER BABIES'

For decades, there have been fears that IVF has the potential to create 'designer babies', where genes are selected to ensure children have certain preferable traits, such as a particular eye colour or a higher IQ. But selecting traits brought about by multiple genes (as opposed to genetic diseases caused by a single mutation) is actually very complicated and may not be possible – at least for the time being.

This was evident from a study published in 2019. The researchers carried out a kind of thought experiment where they used genetic information from real people to model the genetic profiles of hypothetical embryos, with a view to selecting embryos based on traits like a higher IQ. But the computer simulations showed that any advantage was actually minimal.

However, in 2018, a company in the US called Genomic Prediction claimed to be using 'polygenic risk scores' to estimate associations between genes and traits in order to predict which embryos are least likely to have different common diseases. In other words, the metric estimates the likelihood of having a particular trait (such as a specific inherited condition) based on the collection of variants within multiple genes associated with that trait. The idea is to be able to offer patients the chance to eliminate embryos with a high risk of conditions such as diabetes, heart attacks, and a number of types of cancer – as well as identify embryos that are likely to have below average intelligence. The company have said they will only offer the technique to fertility clinics to screen out embryos that might have a very low IQ or a mental disability. But there are concerns that, in the future, some clinic somewhere in the world might start singling out embryos with a high IQ, although one subsequent study suggested that such genetic screening followed by artificial selection would have a negligible impact on improving IQ. And anyway, IQ isn't a good measure of intelligence.

But this has raised the idea that science fiction films like *Gattaca* – where genetic selection ensures children possess the best hereditary traits of their parents – could one day become a reality. The 1932 dystopian novel *Brave New World* described a society, set in 2540, that grew babies in vast vats, engineering them into five tiers of intellect. While this is another intriguing science fiction scenario, who knows what the future holds for IVF and the creation of human life.

## STEM CELLS: MAKING EGGS AND SPERM

Stem cells are cells that can either develop into more cells of the same type or become any kind of cell in the body. Various labs around the world are looking into whether they can use stem cells to create sperm and eggs. Research is in its infancy, but the idea is that regular cells from the human body, such as skin cells, could be transformed into stem cells.

The science isn't there quite yet, though, as it's hard to get stem cells to behave in the right way. In most cells, DNA is packaged into 23 pairs of chromosomes. But sperm and eggs only have one set of 23, because the pairs split up during a process known as 'meiosis'. This is the particularly tricky bit. Scientists in Japan have managed this in mice and created primordial germ cells (PGCs), which are the step before gametes, but the researchers have a way to go before managing to do this with human sperm and eggs.

However, this could well be feasible in the not-too-distant future. So, rather than a woman having to undergo all the drug-taking and egg extraction involved in IVF, or a man having to provide a semen sample, they could simply have a bunch of eggs or sperm made from scraps of their skin.

Dr Cesar says…

'In the foreseeable future, I think we will see a generation of eggs, sperm and embryos from stem cells. This will allow us to treat virtually any type of infertility related to ovarian/testicular failure or egg/sperm quality problems (for example, azoospermia [absence of viable sperm in the semen], advanced maternal age or premature ovarian failure) for which, most of the time, the only realistic alternative nowadays is gamete donation. It is already a reality in animal models [animal testing]. It is very difficult to predict how soon this will become a clinical application, but given how other fields of regenerative medicine have expanded, I would say 10 years.'

## ARTIFICIAL EMBRYOS

Other researchers are going a step further and looking at whether they can create artificial human embryos, without the need for a sperm or an egg at all. In 2017, Cambridge University mixed two types of mouse stem cells and attached them onto a 3D 'scaffold', before leaving them in a tank of chemicals – which was designed to mimic conditions inside the uterus. After four days, the cells had formed a structure resembling a mouse embryo.

More recently, scientists in the US have used human stem cells to make structures that mimic early embryos. Their aim was to study the early stages of embryonic development.

While there are currently no plans to use such artificial embryos for reproduction, this could well change in the future.

## ARTIFICIAL WOMBS

Researchers in the Netherlands have been given the go-ahead to develop a prototype for an artificial uterus (womb). The main aim is to enable premature babies to continue developing in a protected environment outside of their mother's womb. It follows successful animal testing of artificial womb prototypes – the Biobag and the EVE – in the US and Australia. Fertility experts also see the potential for use in IVF for patients who aren't able to carry for a full pregnancy.

## PRE-FERTILISATION SEX SELECTION

Pre-implantation genetic diagnosis (PGD), or pre-implantation genetic testing (PGT-M), is already being used for sex selection in the US to help with 'family balancing' (*see* page 129). (PGD to select the sex of a baby is illegal in the UK and many other countries around the world.)

But scientists are now looking into new ways of sex selection before fertilisation has even taken place. In 2019, scientists in Japan reported they had developed a technique to sort mouse sperm carrying an X chromosome from those carrying a Y chromosome. Males have one Y chromosome and one X chromosome, while females have two X chromosomes. So sperm can be picked to fertilise the egg so that offspring are male (XY) or female (XX). The reality is that it may not be long before this technique creeps into use on human sperm.

Paul Wilson says…

'The only way you can reliably identify embryo sex is through genetic testing – although many scientists have observed that male embryos divide faster than female embryos. And some people's perception of what we can do in the lab is completely removed from reality. We've been asked all manner of questions over the years: "Can you tell if the baby will be intelligent?", "Can you tell whether the baby will be good with music?" and even "Can we avoid the embryos with ginger hair?!"'

## OVERCOMING INFERTILITY

As an alternative to tweaking the genetic material of embryos or creating eggs, sperm or embryos from scratch, scientists are also looking at ways to circumvent infertility in eggs and sperm. Here are just a few of the most interesting bits of research happening in labs around the world…

A study by scientists in the UK managed to create healthy offspring from infertile male mice. As I've mentioned, most girls have two X chromosomes (XX) and boys have an X and a Y chromosome (XY). But about 1 in 500 boys are born with an extra X or Y, leading to either Klinefelter syndrome (XXY, *see* page 39) or Double Y syndrome (XYY). When turning some tissue cells into stem cells, the scientists managed to remove the extra sex chromosome in mice to produce fertile offspring. The hope is that this might be possible in humans in the future.

Other research has focused on a condition known as primary ovarian insufficiency (POI), where women hit the menopause before the age of 40, rendering them infertile. Scientists at Stanford University School of Medicine in the US managed to induce the ovaries to produce eggs in some infertile women with the condition. Cutting the ovaries into pieces was found to wake up dormant cells, meaning that egg supply was conserved, before the eggs were then treated with drugs. The study was only carried out in a small number of women in Japan, but initial results look promising.

Meanwhile, a fertility clinic in Greece claims to have found a way to restart periods in women who have been through menopause. The Genesis Athens clinic says researchers have rejuvenated ovaries using a blood treatment that helps wounds heal faster. By injecting so-called platelet-rich plasma (PRP) into the ovaries of post-menopausal women, the researchers managed to restart periods in around 30 women between the ages of 46 and 49, and collect and fertilise eggs.

From restarting periods to making older eggs young again – a technique pioneered by scientists in the US claims to be able to turn back the clock by adding a fresh set of 'batteries' transferred from more youthful ovarian cells. As mentioned before in this chapter, mitochondria are the 'power stations' of cells. By sucking them out of immature ovarian stem cells and injecting them into mature egg cells, the researchers have managed to give the ageing cells a new lease of life. However, some scientists have questioned whether such stem cells would still exist in ovaries later in life.

And, finally, another study looked at ways to extend a woman's window of fertility. Believe it or not, the microscopic worm *Caenorhabditis elegans* has many of the same genes as humans, including those that drive ageing processes. Researchers at Princeton University in the US used a drug that extended the egg viability in the worm. Developing this for humans would be a big leap but, in the future, it could theoretically be possible to extend a women's fertility.

## AN EVOLVING LANDSCAPE

The landscape of assisted conception is rapidly evolving. Not only is technology becoming ever more advanced, there are now all sorts of personalised services on offer to support you through the whole process. Whether all the developments that we've discussed in this chapter are ultimately beneficial and will become the norm in the future, who knows?

What these developments do is call into question how far we're prepared to go to create life. Certainly, they have raised in my mind questions about how far Max and I would have gone to have a child. If faced with the prospect of one chance at a child who we knew would carry a gene for a serious disease, would we still have decided to go ahead with trying to get pregnant with that embryo? What if there had been the option of gene editing to remove that issue? If everyone else was tweaking genes to 'design' their baby, would we have too?

In 2010, a Vatican official strongly disapproved of one of the IVF pioneers receiving a Nobel Prize. I wonder what he thinks now of gene editing and mitochondrial donation? After all, the backlash against the early pioneers of IVF now seem laughable. So, another 40 years on, will the current disapproving frowns towards 'designer babies' be laughed at, too?

Ethics committees are right to hold tightly to the reins of scientific progress – particularly when it comes to genetic engineering and the quest for the 'perfect child'. There will be many out there who hanker after perfection. But what is perfect? One person's idea of perfection is another's imperfection.

For Max and I, we just feel so lucky to have had our children. IVF enabled us to do this – and for that we'll be eternally grateful.

Dr Valentine says…

'Attitudes not only can change, they do change. When IVF was first available, there were so many people against it. A few decades ago, in this country, it was considered "adoption by proxy" if donor sperm was used. I also remember when using donor sperm with a single woman or same-sex couple was considered inappropriate – yet now it's completely normal, and rightly so. It's staggering to think of how we've moved on. Society changes and things that were *not* acceptable become acceptable.'

# Afterword

Whatever your reason for reading this book, I hope that it has helped. Going through fertility treatment is such a difficult journey, which can be fraught with confusion, unforeseen challenges, extreme emotions and huge financial sacrifice.

If you finally discover why you're struggling to conceive, it can feel like such a relief after months – or even years – in the dark. But finding out what's wrong is just the start. In some cases it can be enough to tweak your diet or lifestyle. In other cases, it's a long, rocky road through treatment and beyond.

Hopefully this book helps to clarify the process of what's involved in going through treatment and explains what the stats and science suggest is worth investing in, while giving advice on how to choose the right clinic and pathway for you, as well as providing support through stressful times regardless of whether treatment is or isn't successful.

While the fertility industry in this country is highly regarded and well regulated by the Human Fertilisation and Embryology Authority (HFEA), this book highlights that there are still issues such as the postcode lottery, and misconceptions about things like add-ons and success rates. But I hope the book will help you see the wood for the trees. It's a manual that I didn't have to hand when I went through IVF.

Everybody's journey is different, with different challenges and outcomes. The main thing to bear in mind is that you're not alone – from consultants to counsellors to confidantes, there are caring professionals and friends and family to help you along the way. Lean on them. And this book is here to provide support for when you can't quite remember what you're doing and why.

Anyone who has been through fertility treatment will have felt lost or confused at times, and experienced a full gamut of emotions from elation to depression, and been niggled by fears and misgivings. You've taken on a tough challenge. So hang on in there. And, crucially, be kind to yourself.

# Glossary

**Add-ons:** Optional additional treatments that you can have on top of standard IVF, such as assisted hatching, embryo glue, endometrial scratch.

**Anti-Müllerian hormone (AMH):** Produced by cells within the ovary, the levels of this hormone give an indication of ovarian reserve.

**Assisted hatching:** When the embryo is helped to 'hatch' using an acidic solution, lasers or other tools to thin or pierce the membrane surrounding the embryo.

**Blastocyst:** A multicellular embryo, five to six days after fertilisation.

**Chromosomes:** Structures inside cells that carry genes and are mostly made of DNA.

**Cryopreservation:** Freezing eggs, sperm or embryos.

**Egg sharing:** When a patient going through IVF donates eggs collected during their treatment.

**Elective freezing:** When a patient decides before starting treatment that after the fertilisation stage, they will freeze all embryos.

**Embryo glue:** A substance that is added to the Petri dish containing the embryo before embryo transfer. The theory is that it may improve the chances of successful embryo implantation.

**Endometrial scratch:** When the endometrium is scraped with a sterile plastic tube before embryo transfer. The theory is that this may cause the body to release chemicals and hormones to repair the scratch site, hence creating the right environment for embryo implantation.

**Endometriosis:** When the uterus lining grows outside the uterus, damaging the ovaries or fallopian tubes.

**Endometrium:** The lining of the uterus (womb), which thickens during the menstrual cycle in preparation for possible embryo implantation.

**Follicle:** A fluid-filled sac in an ovary, which contains an egg.

**Follicle-stimulating hormone (FSH):** Produced by the pituitary gland, follicle-stimulating hormone (FSH) prompts follicles in the ovaries to grow and mature.

**Gamete:** A sperm or an egg.

**Intracytoplasmic sperm injection (ICSI):** A fertility treatment where the partner's (or donor's) sperm is injected directly into an egg, and then the embryo is inserted (transferred) into the uterus (womb).

**In vitro fertilisation (IVF):** A fertility treatment where eggs are extracted from the ovaries, fertilised with the partner's (or donor's) sperm by placing them both in a Petri dish, and then the embryo is inserted (transferred) into the uterus (womb).

**Intra-uterine insemination (IUI):** A fertility treatment where sperm are injected into the uterus using a fine plastic straw and left to fertilise the eggs naturally.

**Luteinising hormone (LH):** Produced by the pituitary gland, luteinising hormone (LH) triggers ovulation in women. (In men, it stimulates the testes to produce testosterone.)

**Menstrual cycle:** A woman's natural reproductive cycle, involving ovulation and menstruation.

**Menstruation:** When blood and other material from the lining of the uterus is discharged about once a month from puberty until the menopause, except during pregnancy. Commonly known as a 'period'.

**Mild stimulation IVF / IVF lite:** A fertility treatment just like a standard antagonist cycle of IVF, where much lower doses of egg-boosting drugs are used.

**Morula:** An early-stage embryo consisting of 16 cells, which forms around three to four days after fertilisation.

**Natural cycle IVF:** A fertility treatment where no fertility drugs are used at all. The one egg released as part of the natural menstrual cycle is mixed with sperm as with standard IVF.

**Natural cycle modified IVF:** A modified form of natural cycle IVF where some fertility drugs are used.

**Oestrogen:** Produced by the endocrine system, this hormone helps to regulate the menstrual cycle, supports foetal development, and regulates the production of other pregnancy hormones.

**Ovary:** A female reproductive organ in which eggs are produced.

**Ovarian hyperstimulation syndrome (OHSS):** When too many follicles or eggs develop in the ovaries, so they swell and become painful.

**Ovarian reserve:** The ability of the ovaries to produce viable eggs from follicles in the ovaries.

**Ovulation:** When an egg is released from a follicle in an ovary.

**Polycystic ovary syndrome (PCOS):** When a woman has ovaries with a large number of follicles that don't release eggs.

**Pre-implantation genetic diagnosis (PGD):** A technique used to check the genes of embryos for a specific genetic condition. Also known as pre-implantation genetic testing (PGT-M).

**Pre-implantation genetic screening (PGS):** A technique that tests embryos to see if they have the normal number of chromosomes.

**Progesterone:** A hormone released by the ovary, which plays important roles in the menstrual cycle and in maintaining the early stages of pregnancy.

**Testosterone:** A hormone that supports sperm production in men.

**Time-lapse imaging:** A machine that captures images of an embryo inside an incubator, removing the need for the embryologist to take the embryo out of the incubator to check it.

**Vitrification:** A technique where eggs, sperm or embryos are frozen at much faster rates than in traditional slow freezing.

**Zona pellucida:** The membrane surrounding an egg.

**Zygote:** A cell formed when a sperm fertilises an egg.

# References

## INTRODUCTION

'around 3.5 million couples are finding it difficult to conceive': Infertility: overview, NHS Direct Wales: https://www.nhsdirect.wales.nhs.uk/Encyclopaedia/i/article/infertility/; Infertility: overview, NHS: https://www.nhs.uk/conditions/infertility/; Fertility conditions, Fertility Network UK: https://fertilitynetworkuk.org/fertility-faqs/fertility-conditions/.

'over 74,000 cycles in 2018/2019': State of the Fertility Sector: 2018–19, HFEA. [Online] Available from: www.hfea.gov.uk/about-us/publications/research-and-data/fertility-treatment-2018-trends-and-figures/; Fertility trends explained, Fertility treatment 2017: trends and figures report, HFEA, published May 2019. [Online] Available from: https://www.hfea.gov.uk/about-us/publications/research-and-data/fertility-trends-explained/.

'$25bn (£19.10bn) has been generated globally from fertility services': (2019) The fertility business is booming, *The Economist*, 8 August 2019. [Online] Available from: https://www.economist.com/business/2019/08/08/the-fertility-business-is-booming.

'already more than 6 million people who were born via IVF': New exhibition opens to celebrate 40 years of IVF, HFEA, 2018. [Online] Available from: https://www.hfea.gov.uk/about-us/news-and-press-releases/2018-news-and-press-releases/new-exhibition-opens-to-celebrate-40-years-of-ivf/.

'3 per cent of the world's population may exist because of assisted reproductive technologies': Faddy, M, Gosden, M, Gosden, R. (2018) A demographic projection of the contribution of assisted reproductive technologies to world population growth, RBMO, April 2018. [Online] Available from: https://www.rbmojournal.com/article/S1472-6483(18)30039-7/fulltext.

'in 2018 the average birth rate per embryo' Available from: www.hfea.gov.uk/about-us/publications/research-and-data/fertility-treatment-2018-trends-and-figures/.

'for women under 35 it was even higher': Fertility trends explained, Fertility treatment 2017: trends and figures report, HFEA, published May 2019. [Online] Available from: https://www.hfea.gov.uk/about-us/publications/research-and-data/fertility-trends-explained/; (2017) IVF more popular, successful and safer than ever but reasons for treatment are changing, Fertility treatment 2017: trends and figures report, HFEA, published May 2019. [Online] Available from: https://www.hfea.gov.uk/about-us/news-and-press-releases/2019-news-and-press-releases/ivf-more-popular-successful-and-safer-than-ever-but-reasons-for-treatment-are-changing/.

'their ovaries hold millions of fluid-filled sacs called follicles': What are ovarian follicles? London Women's Clinic. [Online] Available from: www.londonwomensclinic.com/what-are-follicles-and-why-are-they-important-for-my-fertility/.

'by puberty less than half a million will remain': Akande, V. (2018) Ovarian reserve and fertility changes with age, BCRM, 8 April 2018. [Online] Available from: https://www.fertilitybristol.com/ovarian-reserve-and-fertility/.

'throughout her life she will constantly lose eggs': (2010) Biological clock studied, NHS. [Online] Available from: www.nhs.uk/news/pregnancy-and-child/biological-clock-studied/.

'men constantly produce fresh sperm every day': Tanrikut, C. (2019) The lifecycle of sperm: sperm development, Shady Grove Fertility, 5 June 2019. [Online] Available from: https://www.shadygrovefertility.com/blog/fertility-health/fertility-facts-sperm-regeneration/.

'Sperm take up to three months to fully mature': Tanrikut, C. (2019) The lifecycle of sperm: sperm development, Shady Grove Fertility, 5 June 2019. [Online] Available from: https://www.shadygrovefertility.com/blog/fertility-health/fertility-facts-sperm-regeneration/.

'the sperm use their tails to propel themselves along': Freudenrich, C. and Edmonds, M., How human reproduction works, HowStuffWorks. [Online] Available from: https://health.howstuffworks.com/pregnancy-and-parenting/pregnancy/conception/human-reproduction2.htm.

'there are all sorts of obstacles for sperm to get around': (2009) The Great Sperm Race, Channel 4 documentary, 2009. [Online] Available from: http://www.channel4.com/microsites/G/TGSR/PDF/Great-Sperm-Race.pdf; Martin, R.D. (2017) A sperm's obstacle course to the egg, Psychology Today, 6 September 2017. [Online] Available from: https://www.psychologytoday.com/us/blog/how-we-do-it/201709/sperm-s-obstacle-course-the-egg.

'each male ejaculation releases millions and millions of sperm': Olson, E.R. (2013) Why are 250 million sperm cells released during sex? Live Science, 24 January 2013. [Online] Available from: https://www.livescience.com/32437-why-are-250-million-sperm-cells-released-during-sex.html.

'and the cervical mucus thins to let the sperm pass through': Trying to get pregnant, NHS. [Online] Available from: www.nhs.uk/conditions/pregnancy-and-baby/getting-pregnant/.

'The athletic ones survive there for up to five days': How long do sperm live after ejaculation? Mayo Clinic. [Online] Available from: www.mayoclinic.org/healthy-lifestyle/getting-pregnant/expert-answers/pregnancy/faq-20058504.

'shunt it down the tube, ready for its speed date with sperm': Trying to get pregnant, NHS. [Online] Available from: www.nhs.uk/conditions/pregnancy-and-baby/getting-pregnant/.

'two sperm have been known to penetrate and fertilise the egg simultaneously': (2019) Semi-identical twins 'identified for only the second time', BBC News, 27 February 2019. [Online] Available from: https://www.bbc.co.uk/news/health-47371431.

'within five to six days, it becomes a multi-cellular blastocyst': Blastocyst Culture, Transfer & Implantation, London Women's Clinic. [Online] Available from: www.londonwomensclinic.com/fertility-treatments/blastocyst-culture-implantation/

## CHAPTER 1

'While 80–90 per cent of couples trying for a baby will get pregnant within one year': Trying to get pregnant: Your pregnancy and baby guide. NHS: https://www.nhs.uk/conditions/pregnancy-and-baby/getting-pregnant/; How long does it usually take to get pregnant? NHS: https://www.nhs.uk/common-health-questions/pregnancy/how-long-does-it-usually-take-to-get-pregnant/.

'a quarter of people that seek fertility treatment suffer from 'unexplained infertility'': Infertility: causes. NHS: https://www.nhs.uk/conditions/infertility/causes/.

'where there is no clear reason for not being able to conceive': Getting started: Your guide to fertility treatment, HFEA. [Online] Available from: https://ifqlive.blob.core.

windows.net/umbraco-website/2110/hfea_a5_getting_started_guide_2017_pdf_for_upload_tagged_rev-1.pdf.

'the sperm will have had time to travel up the fallopian tubes': Trying to get pregnant: Your pregnancy and baby guide. NHS: https://www.nhs.uk/conditions/pregnancy-and-baby/getting-pregnant/; How can I tell when I'm ovulating? NHS: https://www.nhs.uk/common-health-questions/womens-health/how-can-i-tell-when-i-am-ovulating/

'Body mass index (BMI) is calculated using your height and weight': What is the body mass index (BMI)? NHS: https://www.nhs.uk/common-health-questions/lifestyle/what-is-the-body-mass-index-bmi/.

'Some viral infections, such as coronaviruses' [Online] Available from: https://www.rcog.org.uk/en/guidelines-research-services/guidelines/coronavirus-pregnancy/covid-19-virus-infection-and-pregnancy/#general.

'as well as levels of anti-Müllerian hormone (AMH)': Ovarian reserve and the chance of success, London Women's Clinic. [Online] Available from: https://www.londonwomensclinic.com/news-section/posts/2018/october/ovarian-reserve-and-the-chance-of-success/.

'Laparoscopy – checks fallopian tubes': Vandergriendt, C. (2017) What to expect from laparoscopy for endometriosis, healthline. [Online] Available from: https://www.healthline.com/health/endometriosis/laparoscopy-for-endometriosis.

'Hysteroscopy – checks for fibroids or': Hysteroscopy: overview, NHS: https://www.nhs.uk/conditions/hysteroscopy/; Getting started: Your guide to fertility treatment, HFEA. [Online] Available from: https://ifqlive.blob.core.windows.net/umbraco-website/2110/hfea_a5_getting_started_guide_2017_pdf_for_upload_tagged_rev-1.pdf.

'Biopsy – analysis of the uterus lining (endometrium)': Biopsy: overview, NHS: https://www.nhs.uk/conditions/biopsy/.

'Thyroid problems … are occasionally to blame for lack of ovulation': Infertility: causes, NHS: https://www.nhs.uk/conditions/infertility/causes/.

'a loss of ovarian function before the age of 40': Premature ovarian insufficiency (POI), Guy's and St Thomas NHS Foundation Trust information sheet. [Online] Available from: https://www.guysandstthomas.nhs.uk/resources/patient-information/gynaecology/premature-ovarian-insufficiency.pdf.

'ovaries with a large number of follicles that don't release eggs': Polycystic ovary syndrome: overview, NHS: https://www.nhs.uk/conditions/polycystic-ovary-syndrome-pcos/.

'Those who do have symptoms may have irregular or non-existent periods': (2018) Polycystic ovary syndrome: Scientists closer to understanding cause, BBC News, 15 May 2018. [Online] Available from: https://www.bbc.co.uk/news/world-44127615; Klein, A. (2018) Cause of polycystic ovary syndrome discovered at last, New Scientist, 14 May 2018. [Online] Available from: https://www.newscientist.com/article/2168705-cause-of-polycystic-ovary-syndrome-discovered-at-last/.

'excessive levels of anti-Müllerian hormone (AMH)': Tata, B. et al (2018) Elevated prenatal anti-Müllerian hormone reprograms the fetus and induces polycystic ovary syndrome in adulthood, Nature Medicine 24, pp. 834–846.

'vital to keep all the cells in your body working normally': Your thyroid gland, British Thyroid Foundation. [Online] Available from: https://www.btf-thyroid.org/what-is-thyroid-disorder.

'both of which interfere with ovulation': Underactive thyroid (hypothyroidism): overview, NHS: https://www.nhs.uk/conditions/underactive-thyroid-hypothyroidism/; Overactive thyroid (hyperthyroidism): overview, NHS: https://www.nhs.uk/conditions/overactive-thyroid-hyperthyroidism/; Thompson, D. (2017) Mild low thyroid levels may affect a woman's fertility, WebMD, 20 December 2017. [Online] Available from: https://www.webmd.com/infertility-and-reproduction/news/20171220/mild-low-thyroid-levels-may-affect-a-womans-fertility#1; (2019) Tobah, Y.B. For women, is there any connection between hypothyroidism and infertility? Mayo Clinic, 13 June 2019. [Online] Available from: https://www.mayoclinic.org/diseases-conditions/female-infertility/expert-answers/hypothyroidism-and-infertility/faq-20058311; Rodriguez, D. (2013) Thyroid issues and fertility: what to know, *Everyday Health*, 21 February 2013. [Online] Available from: https://www.everydayhealth.com/thyroid-conditions/thyroid-issues-and-fertility.aspx.

'cervical surgery can scar the area or shorten the neck of the womb': Infertility: causes, NHS: https://www.nhs.uk/conditions/infertility/causes/.

'Endometriosis can affect fertility, but exactly why isn't yet fully understood – it's thought it could be something to do with the damage to the ovaries or fallopian tubes'. Endometriosis: overview, NHS: https://www.nhs.uk/conditions/endometriosis/.

'Other symptoms include chronic pelvic pain, nausea, constipation or diarrhoea': Endometriosis: overview, NHS: https://www.nhs.uk/conditions/endometriosis/.

'An estimated 176 million women worldwide suffer from the condition': Wood, R. *et al* Myths and misconceptions in endometriosis, endometriosis.org. [Online] Available from: http://endometriosis.org/resources/articles/myths/.

'Your fallopian tubes can be checked and endometriosis identified': (2017) Endometriosis: diagnosis and management, NICE Guideline [NG73], published September 2017. [Online] Available from: https://www.nice.org.uk/guidance/ng73/chapter/Recommendations#endometriosis-symptoms-and-signs; When it's used: Laparoscopy (keyhole surgery), NHS: https://www.nhs.uk/conditions/laparoscopy/why-its-done/.

'there's some success using hormone medicines, or via surgery': Endometriosis: overview, NHS: https://www.nhs.uk/conditions/endometriosis/.

'In England in 2018, 49 per cent of all new STI diagnoses were for chlamydia': Sexually transmitted infections and screening for chlamydia in England, 2018, Public Health England Health Protection Report 13(19), published 7 June 2019. [Online] Available from: https://assets.publishing.service.gov.uk/government/uploads/system/uploads/attachment_data/file/806118/hpr1919_stis-ncsp_ann18.pdf.

'if untreated it can cause all sorts of long-term health problems': (2016) Sexually transmitted infections factsheet, Family Planning Association (FPA), November 2016. [Online] Available from: https://www.fpa.org.uk/factsheets/sexually-transmitted-infections; Chlamydia: overview, NHS: https://www.nhs.uk/conditions/chlamydia/; (2005) Chlamydia and infertility, BBC News, 16 October 2005. [Online] Available from: http://news.bbc.co.uk/1/hi/programmes/panorama/4347858.stm.

'The disease affects both male and female fertility': (2016) Sexually transmitted infections factsheet, Family Planning Association (FPA), November 2016. [Online] Available from: https://www.fpa.org.uk/factsheets/sexually-transmitted-infections.

'This can cause scarring and eventually block the tubes': (2005) Chlamydia and infertility, BBC News, 16 October 2005. [Online] Available from: http://news.bbc.co.uk/1/hi/programmes/panorama/4347858.stm.

'if the fallopian tubes are badly damaged by the disease': (2019) Interview with Dr Kailasam.

'damage to the fallopian tubes *might* be attributable to chlamydia infection': Price, M.J. *et al* (2012) How much tubal factor infertility is caused by Chlamydia? Estimates based on serological evidence corrected for sensitivity and specificity, *Sexually Transmitted Diseases* 39(8), pp. 608–613.

'the probability of tubal infertility': Kavanagh, K. *et al* (2013) Estimation of the risk of tubal factor infertility associated with genital chlamydial infection in women: a statistical modelling study, *International Journal of Epidemiology* 42(2), pp. 493–503.

'Gonorrhoea and mycoplasma also affect fertility': Boskey, E. (2019) Can STDs affect my ability to have children? Verywell Health, 29 November 2019. [Online] Available from: https://www.verywellhealth.com/can-an-std-cause-infertility-3133182.

'One in two people in the UK will be diagnosed with some sort of cancer during their lifetime': Lifetime risk of cancer, Cancer Research UK. [Online] Available from: https://www.cancerresearchuk.org/health-professional/cancer-statistics/risk/lifetime-risk.

'9 per cent of these cancer cases affect people between the ages of 30 and 49': Baker, C. (2016) Cancer statistics: in brief, House of Commons Library Briefing Paper No SN06887, 6 December 2016. [Online] Available from: researchbriefings.files. parliament.uk/documents/SN06887/SN06887.pdf

'they can sometimes cause irreversible damage to the ovaries': Molina, J.R. *et al* (2005) Chemotherapy-induced ovarian failure: manifestations and management, *Drug Safety* 28(5), pp. 401–16; Bedoschi, G. *et al* (2016) Chemotherapy-induced damage to ovary: mechanisms and clinical impact, *Future Oncology* 12(20), pp. 2333–2334; Waimey, K.E. *et al* (2015) Understanding fertility in young cancer patients, *Journal of Women's Health* 24(10), pp. 812–818; How chemotherapy affects women's fertility, Cancer Research UK. [Online] Available from: https://www.cancerresearchuk.org/about-cancer/cancer-in-general/treatment/chemotherapy/fertility/women/how-chemotherapy-affects-fertility.

'Illegal drugs, such as marijuana or cocaine, can mess with ovulation': Shelton, P. (2017) Does marijuana affect fertility? Reproductive Health Center, 17 May 2017. [Online] Available from: https://www.ivftucson.com/marijuana-affect-fertility/

'in the US the birth rate in women aged over 35 had increased': Harris, I.D. *et al* (2011) Fertility and the Aging Male, *Urology* 13(4) pp. e184–90.

'rise in pregnancy rates from 2015 to 2016 were the over-40s': Rudgard, O. (2018) Older mothers on the rise as over-40s become the only group with a rising conception rate, *The Telegraph*, 27 March 2018. [Online] Available from: https://www.telegraph.co.uk/news/2018/03/27/older-mothers-rise-over-40s-become-group-rising-conception-rate/.

'the average IVF patient age in the UK has increased': Fertility treatment 2017: trends and figures report, HFEA, published May 2019. [Online] Available from: https://www.hfea.gov.uk/media/2894/fertility-treatment-2017-trends-and-figures-may-2019.pdf.

'age is the biggest factor affecting fertility': (2018) IVF treatment safer and more successful than ever before, HFEA, 20 December 2018 [Online] Available from: https://www.hfea.gov.uk/about-us/news-and-press-releases/2018-news-and-press-releases/ivf-treatment-safer-and-more-successful-than-ever-before/

'and then rapidly declining from the age of 37': (2014) Female age-related fertility decline, The American College of Obstetricians and Gynecologists Committee Opinion No 589, March 2014. [Online] Available from: https://www.acog.org/Clinical-Guidance-

and-Publications/Committee-Opinions/Committee-on-Gynecologic-Practice/
Female-Age-Related-Fertility-Decline?IsMobileSet=false.

'but by the age of 38 only 75 per cent will': Getting started: Your guide to fertility treatment,
HFEA. [Online] Available from: https://ifqlive.blob.core.windows.net/umbraco-
website/2110/hfea_a5_getting_started_guide_2017_pdf_for_upload_tagged_rev-1.pdf

'A study of university students to find out whether they are aware of this declining fertility':
Prior, E. et al (2018) Fertility facts, figures and future plans: an online survey of
university students, Human Fertility pp. 22(4), pp. 282–290.

'Graph shows percentage of embryo transfers' [Online] Source: Analyses of the National
ART Surveillance System (NASS) data. Written communication with the Division of
Reproductive Health, National Center for Chronic Disease Prevention and Health
Promotion, Centers for Disease Control and Prevention, June 26, 2020.

'higher levels of stress were associated with lower odds of conception': Wesselink, A.K. *et
al* (2018) Perceived stress and fecundability: A preconception cohort study of North
American couples, *American Journal of Epidemiology* 187(12), pp. 2662–2671.

'could be because the stressed couples were having sex less frequently': Wesselink, A.K. *et
al* (2018) Perceived stress and fecundability: A preconception cohort study of North
American couples, *American Journal of Epidemiology* 187(12), pp. 2662–2671.

'results showed that stress didn't affect the chances of becoming pregnant': Maeda, E. *et
al* (2016) Effects of fertility education on knowledge, desires and anxiety among the
reproductive-aged population: findings from a randomized controlled trial, *Human
Reproduction* 31(9) pp. 2051–2060.

'Our findings show that there is no reason for them to fret': Beckford, M. (2011) Stress
does not stop IVF working, *The Telegraph*, 24 February 2011. [Online] Available from:
https://www.telegraph.co.uk/news/health/news/8345177/Stress-does-not-stop-IVF-
working.html.

'although stress itself doesn't affect fertility, your actions in response to stress might do':
Boivin, J. (2011) Emotional distress in infertile women and failure of assisted reproductive
technologies: meta-analysis of prospective psychosocial studies, *BMJ* 2011;342:d223.

'whether stress affects the chances of getting pregnant when specifically going through
fertility treatment': Witkin, G. (2018) The truth about stress and fertility, *Psychology
Today*, 19 March 2018. [Online] Available from: https://www.psychologytoday.com/
gb/blog/the-chronicles-infertility/201803/the-truth-about-stress-and-fertility.

'study of 166 women found no evidence that psychological stress had any influence':
Anderheim, L. *et al* (2005) Does psychological stress affect the outcome of *in vitro*
fertilization? *Human Reproduction* 20(10), pp. 2969–2975.

'cast doubt on the idea that stress inhibits the success of fertility treatment': Nicoloro-
SantaBarbara, J. *et al* (2018) Just relax and you'll get pregnant? Meta-analysis examining
women's emotional distress and the outcome of assisted reproductive technology,
*Social Science & Medicine* 213, pp. 54–62; https://medicalxpress.com/news/2018-07-
women-emotional-distress-poor-infertility.html.

'people who view a demanding situation as *challenging* perform a lot better': Jones, M.
Facing up to the challenges of stress, Staffordshire University Faculty of Health Sciences.
[Online] Available from: https://www.staffs.ac.uk/assets/facing-up-to-stress.pdf.

'average birth rate for women of all ages using their own eggs': IVF more popular, successful
and safer than ever but reasons for treatment are changing, Fertility treatment 2017:
trends and figures report, HFEA, published May 2019. [Online] Available from: https://

www.hfea.gov.uk/about-us/news-and-press-releases/2019-news-and-press-releases/ivf-more-popular-successful-and-safer-than-ever-but-reasons-for-treatment-are-changing/.

'It also makes the brain focus on just the movement': (2018) Exercise and stress: Get moving to manage stress, Mayo Clinic, 8 March 2018. [Online] Available from: https://www.mayoclinic.org/healthy-lifestyle/stress-management/in-depth/exercise-and-stress/art-20044469.

'eating foods high in prebiotics: University of Colorado at Boulder (2017) Dietary prebiotics improve sleep, buffer impacts of stress, says study, ScienceDaily, 25 February 2017. [Online] Available from: https://www.sciencedaily.com/releases/2017/02/170225102123.htm.

'eating lots of fruit and veg each day lowers the risk of stress': (2019) Stress-Proof Your Life, The Scientific Guide to a Healthy Body & Brain, Focus magazine Collection, Vol. 11.

'if you're underweight or overweight you could find it more difficult to conceive':
Panth, M. et al (2018) The influence of diet on fertility and the implications for public health nutrition in the United States, Frontiers in Public Health 6(211).

'Leptin is thought to regulate fat storage in the body, but also to affect reproductive hormones': Silvestris, E. et al (2018) Obesity as disruptor of the female fertility, Reproductive Biology and Endocrinology 16(1) p. 22; Karoutsos, P. et al (2016) Obesity and female fertility: The bridging role of leptin, Journal of Data Mining in Genomics and Proteomics 8(1).

'BMI should ideally lie in the range 19–30 before starting treatment': (2013) RCOG, Fertility: assessment and treatment for people with fertility problems. [Online] Available from: www.nice.org.uk/guidance/cg156/evidence/full-guideline-pdf-188539453

'NHS classifies an adult as a healthy weight if': Obesity: overview, NHS: https://www.nhs.uk/conditions/obesity/

'women with a BMI over 27 were three times less likely to conceive': Grodstein, F. et al (1994) Body mass index and ovulatory infertility, Epidemiology 5(2) pp. 247–250.

'chances of conceiving within a year go down': van der Steeg, J.W. et al (2008) Obesity affects spontaneous pregnancy chances in subfertile, ovulatory women, Human Reproduction 23(2), pp. 324–328.

'a higher risk of losing the baby in early pregnancy': Pandey, S. et al (2010) The impact of female obesity on the outcome of fertility treatment, Journal of Human Reproductive Sciences 3(2), pp. 62–67; Dağ, Z.Ö. and Dilbaz, B. (2015) Impact of obesity on infertility in women, Journal of the Turkish-German Gynaecological Association 16(2), pp. 111–117.

'Otherwise you're condemning a lot of overweight people': Norman, R.J. and Mol, B.W.J. (2018) Successful weight loss interventions before in vitro fertilization: fat chance? Fertility and Sterility 110(4), pp. 581–586.

'In the UK, the woman's BMI must be': IVF provision in Scotland, Fertility Fairness. [Online] Available from: http://www.fertilityfairness.co.uk/nhs-fertility-services/ivf-provision-in-scotland/; Do you qualify for NHS treatment? Complete Fertility Centre. [Online] Available from: https://www.completefertility.co.uk/nhs_criteria.php.

'who had a success rate of 50 per cent': Kirby, J. (2011) Too thin to conceive, women warned, Independent, 21 October 2011. [Online] Available from: https://www.

independent.co.uk/life-style/health-and-families/health-news/too-thin-to-conceive-women-warned-2373894.html.

'build some easy exercise into your day when you're trying to conceive': Sharma, R. *et al* (2013) Lifestyle factors and reproductive health: taking control of your fertility, *Reproductive Biology and Endocrinology* 11(66).

'women who were more active before undergoing treatment': Meng, R. *et al* (2018) Maternal physical activity before IVF/ICSI cycles improves clinical pregnancy rate and live birth rate: a systematic review and meta-analysis, *Reproductive Biology and Endocrinology* (16)11.

'Extreme exercise can interfere with reproductive hormones': Sharma, R. *et al* (2013) Lifestyle factors and reproductive health: taking control of your fertility, *Reproductive Biology and Endocrinology* 11(66).

'frequent and hard physical exercise seems to reduce fertility in young women': (2010) Hard workouts, reduced fertility, Norwegian University of Science and Techology (NTNU). [Online] Available from: https://www.ntnu.edu/news/hard-workouts-reduced-fertility.

'reduced the chance of a live birth by 40 per cent and the embryo not implanting': Sharma, R. *et al* (2013) Lifestyle factors and reproductive health: taking control of your fertility, *Reproductive Biology and Endocrinology* 11(66).

'examined in depth the effects of diet and other lifestyle changes on fertility': https://www.hsph.harvard.edu/jorge-chavarro/; https://www.hsph.harvard.edu/walter-willett/;

(2009) Follow the fertility diet? Harvard Mental Health Letter, May 2009, adapted from *The Fertility Diet* by Jorge E. Chavarro, M.D., Walter C. Willett, M.D. and Patrick J. Skerrett (McGraw-Hill, New York, 2009). [Online] Available from: https://www.health.harvard.edu/diseases-and-conditions/follow-fertility-diet.

'For people trying to get pregnant naturally, the researchers suggest': Chiu, Y.H. *et al* (2018) Diet and female fertility: doctor, what should I eat? *Fertility and Sterility* 110(4), pp. 560–569; Gaskins, A.J. and Chavarro, J.E. (2018) Diet and fertility: a review, *American Journal of Obstetrics and Gynecology* 218(4), pp. 379–389.

'40 per cent more likely to get pregnant if they ate a Mediterranean diet': Vujkovic, M. *et al* (2010) The preconception Mediterranean dietary pattern in couples undergoing in vitro fertilization/intracytoplasmic sperm injection treatment increases the chance of pregnancy, *Fertility and Sterility* 94(6), pp. 2096–2101.

'An Assisted Conception Unit in Greece looked at the diets of women going through their first IVF treatment': (2019) European Society of Human Reproduction and Embryology

Mediterranean diet may help women receiving IVF to achieve successful pregnancies, ScienceDaily, 29 January 2018. [Online] Available from: https://www.sciencedaily.com/releases/2018/01/180129223846.htm.

'Certain fats are a key part of our diet': How can I get more omega-3 into my diet and how much difference will it make to my health? *Trust Me, I'm a Doctor*, BBC. [Online] Available from: https://www.bbc.co.uk/programmes/articles/341ZWQjRVCyky3V5cfFpS4N/how-can-i-get-more-omega-3-into-my-diet-and-how-much-difference-will-it-make-to-my-health.

'The body can't make essential fatty acids': Di Pasquale, M.G. (2009) The essentials of essential fatty acids, *Journal of Dietary Supplements* 6(2), pp. 143–161.

'little evidence that a moderate amount of caffeine has a detrimental effect': Minguez-Alarcón, L. *et al* (2018) Caffeine, alcohol, smoking, and reproductive outcomes among couples undergoing assisted reproductive technology treatments, *Fertility and Sterility* 110(4), pp. 587–592.

'"maternal caffeine consumption has adverse effects on the success rates of assisted reproduction procedures"': (2019) NICE Pathway, In vitro fertilisation treatment for people with fertility problems.

'even moderate amounts can affect whether IVF works or not': Anderson, K. *et al* (2010) Lifestyle factors in people seeking infertility treatment – A review, *Australian and New Zealand Journal of Obstetrics and Gynaecology* 50(1), pp. 8–20.

'A 2017 study on 221 couples undergoing fertility treatment': Van Heertum, K. and Rossi, B. (2017) Alcohol and fertility: how much is too much? *Fertility Research and Practice* 3(10).

'live birth rates were reduced for women who consumed four or more drinks a week': Rossi, B. *et al* (2011) Effect of alcohol consumption on in vitro fertilization, *Obstetrics and Gynecology* 117(1), pp. 136–142.

'excessive drinking increases the levels of certain hormones': Van Heertum, K. and Rossi, B. (2017) Alcohol and fertility: how much is too much? *Fertility Research and Practice* 3(10).

'more than 1 unit of alcohol per day reduces the effectiveness of assisted reproduction procedures': (2017) NICE, Fertility problems: assessment and treatment. [Online] Available from: https://www.nice.org.uk/guidance/cg156/chapter/recommendations.

'non-smokers' fertility was as badly affected by excessive exposure to second-hand smoke': (2018) Smoking and infertility: A committee opinion, Practice Committee of the American Society for Reproductive Medicine, Fertility and Sterility 110(4), pp. 611–618. [Online] Available from: https://www.asrm.org/globalassets/asrm/asrm-content/news-and-publications/practice-guidelines/for-non-members/smoking_and_infertility.pdf.

'Various pieces of research have revealed why this is the case': Wright, K.P. *et al* (2006) The effect of female tobacco smoking on IVF outcomes, *Human Reproduction*, 21(11), pp. 2930–2934.

'smoking adds the equivalent of 10 years to a 20-year-old woman's reproductive age': Lintsen, A.M. *et al* (2005) Effects of subfertility cause, smoking and body weight on the success rate of IVF, *Human Reproduction* 20(7), pp. 1867–1875.

'smoking may advance the time of menopause by up to four years': (2018) Smoking and infertility: A committee opinion, Practice Committee of the American Society for Reproductive Medicine, Fertility and Sterility 110(4), pp. 611–618. [Online] Available from: https://www.asrm.org/globalassets/asrm/asrm-content/news-and-publications/practice-guidelines/for-non-members/smoking_and_infertility.pdf.

'link between mothers that smoke during pregnancy and reduced sperm counts in their male offspring': Lund University (2018) Sperm count 50 percent lower in sons of fathers who smoke, ScienceDaily, 26 November 2018. [Online] Available from: https://www.sciencedaily.com/releases/2018/11/181126105455.htm.

'Smokers require nearly twice the number of cycles to conceive compared to non-smokers': (2018) Smoking and infertility: A committee opinion, Practice Committee of the American Society for Reproductive Medicine, Fertility and Sterility 110(4), pp. 611–618. [Online] Available from: https://www.asrm.org/globalassets/asrm/asrm-content/news-and-publications/practice-guidelines/for-non-members/smoking_and_infertility.pdf.

'smoking reduces the thickness of the endometrium (uterus lining)': Heger, A. *et al* (2018) Smoking decreases endometrial thickness in IVF/ICSI patients, *Geburtshilfe Frauenheilkunde* 78(1), pp. 78–82.

'were 50 per cent more likely to have a baby': Fleming, N. (2006) Smoking 'reduces the changes of pregnancy', *The Telegraph*, 9 November 2006. [Online] Available from: https://www.telegraph.co.uk/news/uknews/1533652/Smoking-reduces-the-chances-of-pregnancy.html.

'the NHS won't fund IVF for anyone who smoke': IVF: availability, NHS: https://www.nhs.uk/conditions/ivf/availability/

'the flavoured solutions may contain harmful contaminants': Rosenfeld. J. (2029) Can vaping impair fertility? *Medical Economics*, 7 October 209. [Online] Available from: https://www.medicaleconomics.com/sexual-health/can-vaping-impair-fertility.

'vaping may harm fertility in young women, because of its effect in mice': (2019) Vaping may harm fertility in young women, EurekAlert!, 5 September 2019. [Online] Available from: https://www.eurekalert.org/pub_releases/2019-09/tes-vmh090319.php.

'success rates were lower for women going through IVF who lived close to major roads': Gaskins, A. *et al* (2018) Residential proximity to major roadways and traffic in relation to outcomes of in vitro fertilization, *Environment International* 115, pp. 239–246.

'lower success rates after IVF if exposed to air pollutants': Legro, R.S. *et al* (2010) Effect of air quality on assisted human reproduction, *Human Reproduction*, 25(5), pp. 1317–1324; (2004) Nitrogen dioxide in the United Kingdom, Air Quality Expert Group, published by DEFRA, 2004. [Online] Available from: https://uk-air.defra.gov.uk/assets/documents/reports/aqeg/nd-summary.pdf.

'caused fertility to decline by 13 per cent': Wetsman, N. (2018) Air pollution might make it harder to get pregnant, *Popular Science*, 14 November 2018. [Online] Available from: https://www.popsci.com/air-pollution-fertility-pregnancy#page-3.

'and so disrupt our reproductive hormones': Carré, J. *et al* (2017) Does air pollution play a role in infertility?: a systematic review, *Environmental Health* 16(82).

'the cause of the problem is related to sperm': Women over 38, HFEA. [Online] Available from: https://www.hfea.gov.uk/i-am/women-over-38/; Agarwal, A. *et al* (2015) A unique view on male infertility around the globe, *Reproductive Biology and Endocrinology*, 13(37).

'Conception success is affected by poor quality sperm': Low sperm count, NHS: https://www.nhs.uk/conditions/low-sperm-count/

'This is caused by conditions such as hypogonadism': Kumar, P. *et al* (2010) Male hypogonadism: Symptoms and treatment, *Journal of Advanced Pharmaceutical Technology and Research* 1(3), pp. 297–301; Male hypogonadism, Mayo Clinic. [Online] Available from: https://www.mayoclinic.org/diseases-conditions/male-hypogonadism/diagnosis-treatment/drc-20354886.

'Between 95 and 99 per cent of men with Klinefelter syndrome are infertile': Klinefelter syndrome, NHS: https://www.nhs.uk/conditions/klinefelters-syndrome/; What are the treatments for symptoms in Klinefelter syndrome (KS)? National Institute of Child Health and Human Development (NICHD). [Online] Available from: https://www.nichd.nih.gov/health/topics/klinefelter/conditioninfo/treatments.

'The STI chlamydia genetically damages the sperm': Khamsi, R. (2007) Chlamydia reduces male fertility by ravaging sperm, *New Scientist*, 15 October 2007. [Online] Available from: https://www.newscientist.com/article/dn12787-chlamydia-reduces-male-fertility-by-ravaging-sperm/.

'If the infection spreads to the testicles and epididymis': Chlamydia: complications, NHS: https://www.nhs.uk/conditions/chlamydia/complications/.

'Mycoplasma and herpes may also affect fertility, but research is minimal': Boskey, E. (2019) Can STDs affect my ability to have children? Verywell Health, 29 November 2019. [Online] Available from: https://www.verywellhealth.com/can-an-std-cause-infertility-3133182.

conceive, it might be worth taking a semen analysis': Low sperm count, NHS: https://www.nhs.uk/conditions/low-sperm-count/

'the average man will ejaculate a volume of around 1.5 millilitres of semen': Rowe, P.J. *et al* (1993) *WHO manual for the standardized investigation and diagnosis of the infertile couple* (World Health Organization, 1993, ISBN: 978 0521431361).

'A low sperm count, known as oligozoospermia': Lower sperm count, NHS: https://www.nhs.uk/conditions/low-sperm-count/

'In the average man, three out of 10 sperm cells have abnormalities': Scheve, T. Understanding the conception process, HowStuffWorks. [Online] Available from: http://health.howstuffworks.com/pregnancy-and-parenting/pregnancy/conception/conception-process.htm.

'at least 4 per cent of the semen sample should have a normal shape': Sperm test, BCRM. [Online] Available from: https://www.fertilitybristol.com/sperm-test/; Rowe, P.J. *et al* (1993) *WHO manual for the standardized investigation and diagnosis of the infertile couple* (World Health Organization, 1993, ISBN: 978 0521431361).

'On average, 40 per cent of sperm are bad swimmers': Scheve, T. Understanding the conception process, HowStuffWorks. [Online] Available from: http://health.howstuffworks.com/pregnancy-and-parenting/pregnancy/conception/conception-process.htm.

'These antibodies are fairly rare': BCRM. [Online] Available from: www.fertilitybristol.com/sperm-test/.

'This condition is known as pyospermia or leukocytospermia': Pyospermia: Overview, Cleveland Clinic. [Online] Available from: https://my.clevelandclinic.org/health/diseases/15220-pyospermia.

'Research has shown that as a man gets older his sperm quality declines': Harris, I.D. *et al* (2011) Fertility and the aging male, *Urology* 13(4) pp. e184–190.

'Male fertility starts to decline around the age of 40 to 45': At what age does fertility begin to decrease? British Fertility Society. [Online] Available from: https://www.britishfertilitysociety.org.uk/fei/at-what-age-does-fertility-begin-to-decrease/.

'five times more likely to take more than a year to conceive': Hassan, M.A. and Killick, S.R. (2003) Effect of male age on fertility: evidence for the decline in male fertility with increasing age, *Fertility and Sterility* 79(3), pp. 1520–1527.

'nearly three times more likely to experience a miscarriage': Columbia University's Mailman School of Public Health (2006) Miscarriage significantly associated with increasing paternal age, ScienceDaily, 3 August 2006. [Online] Available from: https://www.sciencedaily.com/releases/2006/08/060803171027.htm.

'This contrasted starkly with the fertility rate in men under 30': Harris, I.D. *et al* (2011) Fertility and the aging male, *Urology* 13(4) pp. e184–190.

'the average paternal age had risen from 27.4 to 30.9 years old': Bellver, J. and Donnez, J. (2019) Introduction: Infertility etiology and offspring health, *Fertility and Sterility* 111(6), pp. 1033–1035.

'male fertility is affected by obesity': Obesity: overview, NHS: https://www.nhs.uk/conditions/obesity/

'IVF was less likely to work using obese men's sperm': Campbell, J.M. *et al* (2015), Paternal obesity negatively affects male fertility and assisted reproduction outcomes: a systematic review and meta-analysis, *Reproductive BioMedicine Online*, 31(5), pp.593–604.

'an extra 10kg of weight lowered male fertility by 10 per cent': Sim, I-W. and McLachlan, R. (2014) Obesity – a growing issue for male fertility, *Medicine Today*, 15(1), pp. 49–53.

'fish, poultry, whole grains, fruits, vegetables and nuts improves semen quality': Gaskins, A.J. and Chavarro, J.E. (2018), Diet and fertility: a review, *American Journal of Obstetrics and Gynecology*, 18(4), pp. 379–389; Nassan, F.L. *et al* (2018) Diet and men's fertility: does diet affect sperm quality? *Fertility and Sterility* 110(4), pp.570–577; Antioxidants: in depth, National Center for Complementary and Integrative Health. [Online] Available from: https://nccih.nih.gov/health/antioxidants/introduction.htm.

'ate around a couple of handfuls of mixed almonds, hazelnuts and walnuts a day': Therrien, A. (2018) Sperm quality improved by adding nuts to diet, study says, BBC News, 4 July 2018. [Online] Available from: https://www.bbc.co.uk/news/health-44695602.

'men who exercised at least three times a week for an hour': Sharma, R. *et al* (2013) Lifestyle factors and reproductive health: taking control of your fertility, *Reproductive Biology and Endocrinology* 11(66).

'too intense an exercise regime created poorer quality sperm': Vaamonde, D. *et al* (2009) Response of semen parameters to three training modalities, *Fertility and Sterility* 92(6), pp. 1941–1946.

'intense physical activity may affect quality': Jóźków, P. and Rossato, M. (2017), The impact of intense exercise on semen quality, *American Journals of Men's Health* 11(3), pp. 654–662.

'a study at University College London looked at the cycling habits of 5282 men': Hollingsworth, M. *et al* (2014) An observational study of erectile dysfunction, infertility, and prostate cancer in regular cyclists: Cycling for health UK study, *Journal of Men's Health* 11(2); (2014) Cycling does not cause infertility, British scientists find, *The Telegraph*, 7 July 2014. [Online] Available from: https://www.telegraph.co.uk/news/science/science-news/10952228/Cycling-does-not-cause-infertility-British-scientists-find.html.

'found that the exercise may have affected their fertility': Durairajanayagam D. (2018) Lifestyle causes of male infertility, *Arab Journal of Urology*, 16(1), pp. 10–20; Maleki, B.H *et al* (2014) The effects of 16 weeks of intensive cycling training on seminal oxidants and antioxidants in male road cyclists, *Clinical Journal of Sport Medicine* 24(4), pp. 302–307.

'This is also supported by some older studies': Sharma, R. *et al* (2013) Lifestyle factors and reproductive health: taking control of your fertility, *Reproductive Biology and Endocrinology* 11(66); Wise, L.A. *et al* (2011) Physical activity and semen quality among men attending an infertility clinic, *Fertility and Sterility* 95(3), pp. 1025–1030.

'need to be a couple of degrees Celsius cooler than body temperature in order for sperm to develop': Bering, J. (2009) Why do human testicles hang like that? *Scientific American*, 19 November 2009. [Online] Available from: https://blogs.scientificamerican.com/bering-in-mind/why-do-human-testicles-hang-like-that/.

'excessive exposure to heat can kill off germ cells': Durairajanayagam D. (2018) Lifestyle causes of male infertility, *Arab Journal of Urology*, 16(1), pp. 10–20.

'those who wore boxer shorts had a 17 per cent higher sperm count': Sweeney, C. (2018) Boxers or briefs? Loose-fitting underwear may benefit sperm production, Harvard School of Public Health, 8 August 2018. [Online] Available from: https://www.hsph.harvard.edu/news/press-releases/does-underwear-style-affect-sperm-production/; Wong, S. (2018) Tight underwear really is linked to lower sperm counts in men, *New Scientist*, 8 August 2018. [Online] Available from: https://www.newscientist.com/article/2176176-tight-underwear-really-is-linked-to-lower-sperm-counts-in-men/.

'men who kept their phones in their pocket during the day were monitored': (2016) Mobile phones are cooking men's sperm, *The Telegraph*, 22 February 2016. [Online] Available from: https://www.telegraph.co.uk/news/health/news/12167957/Mobile-phones-are-cooking-mens-sperm.html.

'exposure to electromagnetic radiation emitted by mobile phones': Durairajanayagam D. (2018) Lifestyle causes of male infertility, *Arab Journal of Urology*, 16(1), pp. 10–20; Agarwal, A. and Durairajanayagam, D (2015) Are men talking their reproductive health away? Asian Journal of Andrology 17(3) pp. 433–434.

'NICE guidelines recommend men drink no more than 4 units of alcohol a day': (2017) Fertility problems: assessment and treatment NICE Clinical guideline [CG156], published February 2013, updated September 2017. [Online] Available from: https://www.nice.org.uk/guidance/cg156/ifp/chapter/Trying-for-a-baby.

'excessive alcohol consumption affects sperm quality and quantity': Is alcohol harming your fertility? Drinkaware. [Online] Available from: https://www.drinkaware.co.uk/alcohol-facts/health-effects-of-alcohol/fertility-and-pregnancy/is-alcohol-harming-your-fertility/.

'"it makes sense to avoid alcohol altogether"': Sample, I. (2009) Alcohol hinders having a baby through IVF, couples warned, *The Guardian*, 20 October 2009. [Online] Available from: https://www.theguardian.com/lifeandstyle/2009/oct/20/alcohol-hinders-baby-ivf.

'lowered their chances of getting pregnant by more than a quarter': Sample, I. (2009) Alcohol hinders having a baby through IVF, couples warned, *The Guardian*, 20 October 2009. [Online] Available from: https://www.theguardian.com/lifeandstyle/2009/oct/20/alcohol-hinders-baby-ivf.

'the effect of drinking up to 8 units of alcohol per week, seven days before a semen analysis': Fullston, T. *et al* (2017) The most common vices of men can damage fertility and the health of the next generation, *Journal of Endocrinology* 234(2), pp. 1–6.

'drinking a moderate amount of alcohol might boost male fertility': Wiley (2018) Moderate alcohol consumption may boost male fertility, ScienceDaily, 18 July 2018. [Online] Available from: https://www.sciencedaily.com/releases/2018/07/180718082212.htm.

'excessive boozing or binge drinking should be avoided': Fullston, T. *et al* (2017) The most common vices of men can damage fertility and the health of the next generation, *Journal of Endocrinology* 234(2), pp. 1–6; Lucia, D. and Moritz, K. (2017) It's not just mums who need to avoid alcohol when trying for a baby, The Conversation, 6 November 2017. [Online] Available from: https://theconversation.com/its-not-just-mums-who-need-to-avoid-alcohol-when-trying-for-a-baby-83794.

'smoking is bad news for male fertility': Beal, M.A. *et al* (2017) From sperm to offspring: Assessing the heritable genetic consequences of paternal smoking and potential public health impacts, *Mutation Research* 773, pp. 26–50; Mostafa, T. (2010) Cigarette smoking and male infertility, *Journal of Advanced Research* 1(3), pp. 179–186; Donkin, I. and Barrès, R. (2018) Sperm epigenetics and influence of environmental factors, *Molecular Metabolism* 14, pp. 1–11; American Association for Cancer Research (2007) Cigarette smoking alters DNA in sperm, genetic damage could pass to offspring, ScienceDaily, 1 June 2007. [Online] Available from: https://www.sciencedaily.com/releases/2007/06/070601072219.htm;

Gunes, S. *et al* (2018) Smoking-induced genetic and epigenetic alterations in infertile men, *Andrologia* 50(9), p. e13124.

'paternal smoking was linked with significantly lower success rates for IVF': Kovac, J.R. *et al* (2015) The effects of cigarette smoking on male fertility, *Postgraduate Medicine* 127(3), pp. 338–341.

'the sons of fathers who smoked while their partner was pregnant had half as many sperm': Lund University (2018) Sperm count 50 percent lower in sons of fathers who smoke, ScienceDaily, 26 November 2018. [Online] Available from: https://www.sciencedaily.com/releases/2018/11/181126105455.htm; Everett, G. (2018) Sperm counts halved in sons of smoking dads, BioNews, 3 December 2018. [Online] Available from: https://www.bionews.org.uk/page_140111.

'the NHS won't fund IVF treatment for anyone who smokes': IVF: availability, NHS: https://www.nhs.uk/conditions/ivf/availability/

'several electronic cigarette flavours may damage male fertility': (2017) Plea for ban on vaping flavours that harm sperm. [Online] Available from: www.thetimes.co.uk/edition/news/plea-for-ban-on-vaping-flavours-that-harm-sperm-g8pjf5g8h

'taken an illicit drug in the last year': Statistics on drug misuse: England, 2018, NHS Digital, published 7 February 2018. [Online] Available from: https://digital.nhs.uk/data-and-information/publications/statistical/statistics-on-drug-misuse/2018.

'all affected reproductive hormones or sperm in various ways': Sansone, A. *et al* (2018) Smoke, alcohol and drug addiction and male infertility, *Reproductive Biology and Endocrinology* 16(3).

'just under half of all men who get mumps-related orchitis experience some shrinkage of their testicles': Mumps: complications, NHS: https://www.nhs.uk/conditions/mumps/complications/.

'worth getting any symptoms checked out by your GP': Infertility: causes, NHS: https://www.nhs.uk/conditions/infertility/causes/

'men hoping to have a family are often advised to freeze sperm before undergoing chemotherapy': Chemotherapy side effects: fertility and pregnancy, The Royal Marsden NHS Foundation Trust. [Online] Available from: https://www.royalmarsden.nhs.uk/your-care/treatments/chemotherapy/chemotherapy-effects-and-side-effects/fertility-pregnancy.

'BPA (Bisphenol-A) is a plastic embedded in all sorts of everyday items': Bienkowski, B. (2016) Undergoing fertility treatment? Watch your plastics, *Scientific American*, 14 March 2016. [Online] Available from: https://www.scientificamerican.com/article/undergoing-fertility-treatment-watch-your-plastics/.

'80 per cent of teenagers from various schools across Devon had traces of BPA': Exposure to chemical found in plastics 'hard to avoid' in everyday life. [Online] Available from: https://www.exeter.ac.uk/news/featurednews/title_638539_en.html.

'study in Taiwan on 6475 men found that polluting particles affected sperm shape and size': Lao, X.Q. *et al* (2018) Exposure to ambient fine particulate matter and semen quality in Taiwan, *Occupational and Environmental Medicine* 75(2), pp. 148–154.

'two separate studies also revealed the effect of air pollution': Checa Vizcaíno, M.A. et al (2016) Outdoor air pollution and human infertility: a systematic review, Fertility and Sterility 106(4), pp. 897–904.

'while another showed higher sperm DNA fragmentation in steel plant workers': Bosco, L. et al (2018) Sperm DNA fragmentation: An early and reliable marker of air pollution. [Online] Available from: www.ncbi.nlm.nih.gov/pubmed/29448163.

'what you were exposed to when you were in your mother's womb': Interview with Allan Pacey

'for this to translate into the number of eggs a girl is born with being reduced': (2016) Painkiller study examines use in pregnancy, University of Edinburgh News. [Online] Available from: https://www.ed.ac.uk/news/2016/painkillers-270115.

'if one partner changes their lifestyle for more healthy behaviours': Jackson, S.E. *et al* (2015) The influence of partner's behavior on health behavior change: the English longitudinal study of ageing, *JAMA Internal Medicine* 175(3), pp. 385–392.

## CHAPTER 2

'but this time frame depends on how you respond to the drugs': The stages of IVF treatment, Saint Mary's Assisted Reproductive Treatment. [Online] Available from: https://manchesterivf.co.uk/journey/the-stages-of-ivf-treatment.

'here's a general outline of the steps you're likely to go through once you've chosen a clinic': IVF: What happens. NHS. [Online] Available from: https://www.nhs.uk/conditions/ivf/what-happens/.

'The tests for the woman may include': Getting started: Your guide to fertility treatment, HFEA. [Online] Available from: https://ifqlive.blob.core.windows.net/umbraco-website/2110/hfea_a5_getting_started_guide_2017_pdf_for_upload_tagged_rev-1.pdf

'Producing a sperm sample can be quite a challenging moment': Producing a semen sample for analysis, leaflet from UK Professional Fertility Societies. [Online] Available from: https://www.poole.nhs.uk/pdf/Leaflet-Producing.pdf.

'Voltage is gradually ramped up until ejaculation occurs': Electroejaculation, Weill Cornell Medicine Center for Male Reproductive Medicine and Microsurgery. [Online] Available from: http://www.maleinfertility.org/procedures/electroejaculation.

'What's the next step?': Getting started: Your guide to fertility treatment, HFEA. [Online] Available from: https://ifqlive.blob.core.windows.net/umbraco-website/2110/hfea_a5_getting_started_guide_2017_pdf_for_upload_tagged_rev-1.pdf

'if you're happy for your identifying information to be shared': Getting started: Your guide to fertility treatment, HFEA. [Online] Available from: https://ifqlive.blob.core.windows.net/umbraco-website/2110/hfea_a5_getting_started_guide_2017_pdf_for_upload_tagged_rev-1.pdf

'no treatment in addition to the primary treatment has been shown to be definitively advantageous': Segev, Y. *et al* (2010) Is there a place for adjuvant therapy in IVF? *Obstetrical and Gynecological Survey* 65(4), pp. 260–272.

'no significant benefits of acupuncture to improve outcomes of IVF': Qu, F. *et al* (2012) Effects of acupuncture on the outcomes of in vitro fertilization: a systematic review and meta-analysis, *Journal of Alternative and Complementary Medicine* 18(5), pp. 429–439.

'does not provide sufficient evidence that acupuncture improves IVF clinical pregnancy rate': El-Toukhy, T. *et al* (2008), A systematic review and meta-analysis of acupuncture in in vitro fertilisation, *BJOG* 115(10), pp. 1203–1213.

'These findings do not support the use of acupuncture to improve the rate of live births': Smith, C.A. *et al* (2018) Effect of acupuncture vs sham acupuncture on live births among women undergoing in vitro fertilization: a randomized clinical trial, *JAMA Internal Medicine* 319(19), pp. 1990–1998.

'your clinic may recommend using certain fertility drugs before, during and/or after treatment':Getting started: Your guide to fertility treatment, HFEA [Online] Available from: https://ifqlive.blob.core.windows.net/umbraco-website/2110/hfea_a5_getting_ started_guide_2017_pdf_for_upload_tagged_rev-1.pdf.

'gonadotropins can be taken to produce more sperm': Low sperm count, NHS: https:// www.nhs.uk/conditions/low-sperm-count/.

'block the hormone that causes the eggs to be released': Prevention of ovulation, Hull IVF. [Online] Available from: https://www.hullivf.org.uk/treatments/ivf-treatment-steps/ prevention-of-ovulation/.

'and so is used to control the timing of the menstrual cycle': Wardle, P.G. *et al* (1986) Norethisterone treatment to control timing of IVF, *Human Reproduction* 1(7), pp. 455–457.

'As the drugs above affect your progesterone levels' [Online] Available from: https:// www.reproductivefacts.org/news-and-publications/patient-fact-sheets-and-booklets/ documents/fact-sheets-and-info-booklets/progesterone-supplementation-during-in-vitro-fertilization-ivf-cycles/

'in the form of a daily injection or as a nasal spray five times a day': IVF, BCRM. [Online] Available from: https://www.fertilitybristol.com/fertility-treatment/ivf-icsi/.

'the naturally occurring female hormones FSH (follicle-stimulating hormone) and LH (luteinising hormone)': Menopur® 751U Information for the user. [Online] Available from: https://www.medicines.org.uk/emc/files/pil.1294.pdf.

'FSH prompts follicles to mature, while LH stimulates the most developed follicle to release an egg': FSH and LH in females and males, course in Molecular and Cell Biology, University of California, Berkeley: https://mcb.berkeley.edu/courses/mcb135e/fsh-lh. html.

Ovarian hyperstimulation syndrome, *Journal of Human Reproductive Sciences* 4(2), pp. 70–75; Ovarian hyperstimulation syndrome: Overview. Mayo Clinic. [Online] Available from: https://www.mayoclinic.org/diseases-conditions/ovarian-hyperstimulation-syndrome-ohss/symptoms-causes/syc-20354697.

'Any problems usually settle down within a few days': BCRM notes

'Mild OHSS is fairly common and occurs in about 33 per cent of patients: (2016) Ovarian hyperstimulation syndrome, Royal College of Obstetricians and Gynaecologists 'Information for you', published July 2016. [Online] Available from: https://www.rcog. org.uk/globalassets/documents/patients/patient-information-leaflets/gynaecology/ pi_ohss.pdf.

'reduce high levels of the hormone prolactin, which can mess with the production of FSH': Getting started: Your guide to fertility treatment, HFEA [Online] Available from: https://ifqlive.blob.core.windows.net/umbraco-website/2110/hfea_a5_getting_started_guide_2017_pdf_for_upload_tagged_rev-1.pdf.

'a patient might have to be hospitalised in order to be monitored': Ovarian hyperstimulation syndrome: Ovarian hyperstimulation syndrome: Diagnosis. Mayo Clinic. [Online] Available from: https://www.mayoclinic.org/diseases-conditions/ovarian-hyperstimulation-syndrome-ohss/diagnosis-treatment/drc-20354703.

'off the back of a concern that severe cases were being underreported': Ovarian hyperstimulation syndrome, HFEA, report of meeting 24 January 2018. [Online] Available from: https://www.hfea.gov.uk/media/2463/january-2018-ovarian-hyperstimulation-syndrome.pdf.

'The Office for National Statistics recorded two deaths from OHSS': (2018) Number of deaths from Ovarian Hyperstimulation Syndrome (OHSS) registered in England and Wales, 2001 to 2016, release date 5 June 2018: https://www.ons.gov.uk/peoplepopulationandcommunity/birthsdeathsandmarriages/deaths/adhocs/008533numberofdeathsfromovarianhyperstimulationsyndromeohssregisteredinenglandandwales2001to2016.

'the key thing is the quality of each egg': Kerecsenyi, P. (2016) What are follicles & why are they important in IVF? Manchester Fertility, 15 January 2016, updated 24 September 2019. [Online] Available from: https://www.manchesterfertility.com/blog/item/follicles-for-ivf-what-are-follicles-and-how-many-follicles-do-you-need/.

'around 100,000 sperm are placed with the egg in the Petri dish': BCRM personal information meeting.

'pipettes that are just 1mm in diameter to pick up and manoeuvre the developing embryos': BCRM personal information meeting.

'This is around a tenth of a millimetre in diameter': How do embryos survive the freezing process, Scientific American, 13 June 2005. [Online] Available from: https://www.scientificamerican.com/article/how-do-embryos-survive-th/.

'a clear mass of cells inside': BCRM personal information meeting.

'the longer the embryos can develop in the lab, the greater the chance at a pregnancy': de los Santos, M.J. et al (2003) Implantation rates after two, three or five days of embryo culture, Placenta 24 (Suppl B):S13–9.

'chances of pregnancy increase by 10 per cent each day the eggs remain in the incubator post fertilisation': BCRM personal information meeting.

'screening them for genes linked to the genetic condition': Pre-implantation genetic diagnosis (PGD), HFEA. [Online] Available from: https://www.hfea.gov.uk/treatments/embryo-testing-and-treatments-for-disease/pre-implantation-genetic-diagnosis-pgd/.

'embryos without faulty genes can then either be frozen or transferred to the uterus': Seidel, G. (2018) How a scientist says he made a gene-edited baby – and what health worries may ensue, The Conversation, 29 November 2018. [Online] Available from: https://theconversation.com/how-a-scientist-says-he-made-a-gene-edited-baby-and-what-health-worries-may-ensue-107764; https://emedicine.medscape.com/article/273415-overview.

'identification of serious inherited conditions has risen in recent years': Fertility treatment 2017: trends and figures report, HFEA, published May 2019. [Online] Available from: https://www.hfea.gov.uk/media/2894/fertility-treatment-2017-trends-and-figures-may-2019.pdf.

'there's no point in doing an embryo transfer if the endometrium is less than 5mm thick': NICE. [Online] Available from: www.nice.org.uk/donotdo/replacement-of-embryos-into-a-uterine-cavity-with-an-endometrium-of-less-than-5-mm-thickness-is-unlikely-to-result-in-a-pregnancy-and-is-therefore-not-recommended.

'The number of embryos transferred usually depends on your age': See doc in Sources titled 'fertility-embryo-transfer-strategies-during-in-vitro-fertilisation-treatment'; Commissioning guidance for fertility treatment, HFEA [Online] Available from: https://www.hfea.gov.uk/media/2920/commissioning-guidance-may-2019-final-version.pdf.

'just over a 60 per cent success rate with single blastocyst transfer': BCRM personal information meeting.

'transferring two embryos – one of good quality and one poor – cut the chances of getting pregnant': (2017) IVF pregnancy less successful with two embryos, study finds, *The Guardian*, 5 January 2017. Available from https://www.theguardian.com/science/2017/jan/05/ivf-pregnancy-less-successful-with-two-embryos-study-finds.

'the HFEA discourages multiple pregnancies (twins, triplets or more)': Our campaign to reduce multiple births, HFEA [Online] Available from: https://www.hfea.gov.uk/about-us/our-campaign-to-reduce-multiple-births/;

Multiple pregnancy: having more than one baby, Royal College of Obstetricians and Gynaecologists 'Information for you', published November 2016. [Online] Available from:

https://www.rcog.org.uk/globalassets/documents/patients/patient-information-leaflets/pregnancy/pi-multiple-pregnancy.pdf.

'multiple births have dropped': Fertility treatment 2017: trends and figures, HFEA. [Online] Available from: https://www.hfea.gov.uk/media/2894/fertility-treatment-2017-trends-and-figures-may-2019.pdf

'resting for more than 20 minutes after embryo transfer doesn't improve your chances': NICE. [Online] Available from: www.nice.org.uk/donotdo/women-should-be-informed-that-bed-rest-of-more-than-20-minutes-duration-following-embryo-transfer-does-not-improve-the-outcome-of-ivf-treatment.

'it's the male sperm that causes the problem': Intracytoplasmic sperm injection (ICSI), HFEA. [Online] Available from: https://www.hfea.gov.uk/treatments/explore-all-treatments/intracytoplasmic-sperm-injection-icsi/.

'The egg membrane then immediately closes up the hole pierced by the needle': BCRM Personal Information Meeting.

'as with IVF, there are still many other factors affecting a successful pregnancy': Intracytoplasmic sperm injection (ICSI), HFEA. [Online] Available from: https://www.hfea.gov.uk/treatments/explore-all-treatments/intracytoplasmic-sperm-injection-icsi/.

'it's currently slightly more expensive than standard IVF': Intracytoplasmic sperm injection (ICSI), HFEA. [Online] Available from: https://www.hfea.gov.uk/treatments/explore-all-treatments/intracytoplasmic-sperm-injection-icsi/.

'12.9 per cent get pregnant when using fertility drugs': Getting started: Your guide to fertility treatment, HFEA. [Online] Available from: https://ifqlive.blob.core.windows.net/umbraco-website/2110/hfea_a5_getting_started_guide_2017_pdf_for_upload_tagged_rev-1.pdf

'which can be confused with being pregnant': Akande, V. (2016) The 2 week wait following IVF treatment, BCRM, 9 May 2016. [Online] Available from: https://www.

fertilitybristol.com/the-2-week-wait-following-ivf-treatment/; Getting started: Your guide to fertility treatment, HFEA [Online] Available from: https://ifqlive.blob.core. windows.net/umbraco-website/2110/hfea_a5_getting_started_guide_2017_pdf_for_ upload_tagged_rev-1.pdf.

'Your clinic will be able to advise you on this': Intrauterine insemination (IUI), HFEA. [Online] Available from: https://www.hfea.gov.uk/treatments/explore-all-treatments/ intrauterine-insemination-iui/.

'The benefits of IUI…': Intrauterine insemination (IUI), HFEA. [Online] Available from: https://www.hfea.gov.uk/treatments/explore-all-treatments/intrauterine-insemination-iui/.

'success rates are around a third of that for IVF': Intrauterine insemination (IUI), HFEA. [Online] Available from: https://www.hfea.gov.uk/treatments/explore-all-treatments/ intrauterine-insemination-iui/.

'the chances of success depend on the woman's age, the sperm quality and the reasons for low fertility': Intrauterine insemination (IUI), HFEA. [Online] Available from: https:// www.hfea.gov.uk/treatments/explore-all-treatments/intrauterine-insemination-iui/.

'After a number of attempts': Custers, I.M. *et al* (2008) Intrauterine insemination: how many cycles should we perform? *Human Reproduction* 23(4), pp. 885–888.

'this is the one you release naturally during ovulation': HFEA Getting started: Your guide to fertility treatment. [Online] Available from: https://ifqlive.blob.core.windows. net/umbraco-website/2110/hfea_a5_getting_started_guide_2017_pdf_for_upload_ tagged_rev-1.pdf.

'your body won't have to take a break after IVF, so you can try again sooner': IVF options, HFEA. [Online] Available from: https://www.hfea.gov.uk/treatments/explore-all-treatments/ivf-options/.

'the latest stats show it's around 7.5 per cent lower for all ages': IVF options, HFEA. [Online] Available from: https://www.hfea.gov.uk/treatments/explore-all-treatments/ ivf-options/.

'at the moment, Natural Cycle IVF is not recommended by … NICE': IVF options, HFEA. [Online] Available from: https://www.hfea.gov.uk/treatments/explore-all-treatments/ ivf-options/.

'Success rates are slightly higher than with Natural Cycle IVF': Natural modified IVF, Create Fertility. [Online] Available from: https://www.createfertility.co.uk/fertility-treatments/natural-modified-ivf.

'HFEA currently doesn't have any stats on success rates of mild stimulation IVF': IVF options, HFEA. [Online] Available from: https://www.hfea.gov.uk/treatments/explore-all-treatments/ivf-options/.

'for women undergoing IVF where more than 15 eggs are collected': Steward, R.G. *et al* (2014) Oocyte number as a predictor for ovarian hyperstimulation syndrome and live birth: an analysis of 256,381 in vitro fertilization cycles, *Fertility and Sterility* 101(4), pp. 967–973.

'a higher risk of your baby being born early or underweight': Sunkara, S.K. *et al* (2015) Increased risk of preterm birth and low birthweight with very high number of oocytes following IVF: an analysis of 65 868 singleton live birth outcomes, *Human Reproduction* 30(6), pp. 1473–1480.

'a higher risk that your baby will be born early or underweight': Shashikant, M. *et al* (2018) Perinatal outcomes after stimulated versus natural cycle IVF: a systematic review and meta-analysis, *Reproductive BioMedicine Online*, 36(1), pp. 94–101.

'if you use mild stimulation for every patient you will get poorer pregnancy rates and lower chances of having a baby': Zhang, J.J. *et al* (2016) Minimal stimulation IFV vs conventional IVF: a randomized controlled trial, *American Journal of Obstetrics and Gynecology* 214(1) pp. 96.e1–8; Sunkara, S.K. (2011) Association between the number of eggs and live birth in IVF treatment: an analysis of 400 135 treatment cycles, *Human Reproduction* 26(7), pp.1768–1774; Drakopoulos, P. *et al* (2016) Conventional ovarian stimulation and single embryo transfer for IVF/ICSI. How many oocytes do we need to maximize cumulative live birth rates after utilization of all fresh and frozen embryos? *Human Reproduction* 31(2), pp. 370–376; Orvieto, R. *et al* (2017) The myths surrounding mild stimulation in vitro fertilization (IVF), *Reproductive Biology and Endocrinology* 15(1), p.48.

'immature eggs are collected from your ovaries and allowed to mature in the lab': IVF options, HFEA. [Online] Available from: https://www.hfea.gov.uk/treatments/explore-all-treatments/ivf-options/.

'the HFEA only have records of 13 cycles of IVM': IVF options, HFEA. [Online] Available from: https://www.hfea.gov.uk/treatments/explore-all-treatments/ivf-options/.

'each clinic should have at least one person who is trained in infertility counselling': IVF: Support. NHS. [Online] Available from: https://www.nhs.uk/conditions/ivf/support/; HFEA Code of Practice 9th Edition, published October 2018. [Online] Available from: https://www.hfea.gov.uk/media/2565/hfea-draft-code-of-practice-9th-edition-consultation-version.pdf.

'directory of accredited private therapists': IVF: support. NHS: https://www.nhs.uk/conditions/ivf/support/; Getting emotional support, HFEA. [Online] Available from: https://www.hfea.gov.uk/treatments/explore-all-treatments/getting-emotional-support/.

## CHAPTER 3

'When making your decision, there are important factors to consider': Getting started: Your guide to fertility treatment, HFEA. [Online] Available from: https://ifqlive.blob.core.windows.net/umbraco-website/2110/hfea_a5_getting_started_guide_2017_pdf_for_upload_tagged_rev-1.pdf.

'At time of writing this book, there were 134 fertility clinics in the UK': State of the fertility sector 2018/19, HFEA. [Online] Available from: https://www.hfea.gov.uk/media/2974/state-of-the-fertility-sector-2018-19.pdf.

'nearly 60 per cent of patients are having to pay for their treatment': Joanne Triggs talk at RCOG Fertility Forum.

'the average cost of one cycle of IVF is around £5000': In vitro fertilisation, HFEA [Online] Available from: https://www.hfea.gov.uk/treatments/explore-all-treatments/in-vitro-fertilisation-ivf/.

'over three-quarters (77 per cent) of patients who had add-ons': Pilot national fertility patient survey 2018, HFEA. [Online] Available from: https://www.hfea.gov.uk/media/2702/pilot-national-fertility-patient-survey-2018.pdf.

'payment packages or money-back guarantees' https://www.gcrm.co.uk/prices/finance-and-refund-packages/; https://www.accessfertility.com

'A breakdown of some of the treatment fees (as of 2020) at the Bristol Centre for Reproductive Medicine (BCRM)': Affordable treatment with no hidden costs, BCRM: https://www.fertilitybristol.com/faqs-costs/costs/.

'worth looking into what services are on offer': Getting started: Your guide to fertility treatment, HFEA. [Online] Available from: https://ifqlive.blob.core.windows.net/umbraco-website/2110/hfea_a5_getting_started_guide_2017_pdf_for_upload_tagged_rev-1.pdf.

'If the woman turns 40 while undergoing treatment, that cycle can be completed': New NICE guidelines for NHS fertility treatment, NHS, 20 February 2013. [Online] Available from: https://www.nhs.uk/news/pregnancy-and-child/new-nice-guidelines-for-nhs-fertility-treatment/.

'more cycles of IVF led to higher success rates': Chambers, G.M. *et al* (2017) Assisted reproductive technology in Australia and New Zealand: cumulative live birth rates as measures of success, *The Medical Journal of Australia* 207(3), pp. 114–118.

'provided they have never had IVF before and don't suffer from a low ovarian reserve': New NICE guidelines for NHS fertility treatment, NHS, 20 February 2013. [Online] Available from: https://www.nhs.uk/news/pregnancy-and-child/new-nice-guidelines-for-nhs-fertility-treatment/.

'should be offered six cycles of IUI before IVF is considered': New NICE guidelines for NHS fertility treatment, NHS, 20 February 2013. [Online] Available from: https://www.nhs.uk/news/pregnancy-and-child/new-nice-guidelines-for-nhs-fertility-treatment/; fertility-in-vitro-fertilisation-treatment-for-people-with-fertility-problems (see pdf attached to email).

'individual NHS clinical commissioning groups (CCGs) have the final say': IVF: availability, NHS: https://www.nhs.uk/conditions/ivf/availability/

'where you live affects the number of cycles you are offered free on the NHS': Number of CCGs offering 3 IVF cycles has halved since 2013, Fertility Fairness, 30 October 2017: http://www.fertilityfairness.co.uk/number-of-ccgs-offering-3-ivf-cycles-has-halved-since-2013/.

'the number of CCGs offering the recommended three IVF cycles to women under 40 had halved': Number of CCGs offering 3 IVF cycles has halved since 2013, Fertility Fairness, 30 October 2017: http://www.fertilityfairness.co.uk/number-of-ccgs-offering-3-ivf-cycles-has-halved-since-2013/.

'in Scotland an eligible female partner can receive three free cycles if under 40': IVF provision in Scotland, Fertility Fairness: https://www.fertilityfairness.co.uk/nhs-fertility-services/ivf-provision-in-scotland/.

'in Wales it's two cycles for women under 40': IVF provision in Wales, Fertility Fairness: https://www.fertilityfairness.co.uk/nhs-fertility-services/ivf-provision-in-wales/.

'in Northern Ireland it's just one cycle for those under 40': IVF provision in Northern Ireland, Fertility Fairness: https://www.fertilityfairness.co.uk/nhs-fertility-services/ivf-provision-in-northern-ireland/.

'the number of CCGs providing *one* NHS-funded cycle has gone up to 61 per cent': Number of CCGs offering 3 IVF cycles has halved since 2013, Fertility Fairness, 30

October 2017: http://www.fertilityfairness.co.uk/number-of-ccgs-offering-3-ivf-cycles-has-halved-since-2013/.

'For most women, transferring one single embryo is just as successful as transferring two': Finding the best fertility clinic for you, HFEA [Online] Available from: https://www.hfea.gov.uk/choose-a-clinic/finding-the-best-fertility-clinic-for-you/

'multiple births ... are the single greatest health risk to both mothers and babies': Finding the best fertility clinic for you, HFEA. [Online] Available from: https://www.hfea.gov.uk/choose-a-clinic/finding-the-best-fertility-clinic-for-you/; Multiple pregnancy: having more than one baby, Royal College of Obstetricians and Gynaecologists 'Information for you', published November 2016 [Online] Available from: https://www.rcog.org.uk/globalassets/documents/patients/patient-information-leaflets/pregnancy/pi-multiple-pregnancy.pdf

'the risk of the mother dying during childbirth is 2.5 times higher than average': Finding the best fertility clinic for you, HFEA. [Online] Available from: https://www.hfea.gov.uk/choose-a-clinic/finding-the-best-fertility-clinic-for-you/; Commissioning guidance for fertility treatment, HFEA. [Online] Available from: https://www.hfea.gov.uk/media/2920/commissioning-guidance-may-2019-final-version.pdf.

'the HFEA have a policy that only 10 per cent of IVF births should be multiple births': Commissioning guidance for fertility treatment, HFEA. [Online] Available from: https://www.hfea.gov.uk/media/2920/commissioning-guidance-may-2019-final-version.pdf.

'the HFEA has given assisted hatching a red light': Treatment add-ons, HFEA. [Online] Available from: https://www.hfea.gov.uk/treatments/explore-all-treatments/treatment-add-ons/.

'Embryos need to implant in the wall of the uterus': Hammadeh, M.E. *et al* (2011), Assisted hatching in assisted reproduction: a state of the art, *Journal of Assisted Reproduction and Genetics* 28, pp. 119–128.

'scraping the endometrium with a sterile plastic tube before embryo transfer': Treatment add-ons, HFEA. [Online] Available from: https://www.hfea.gov.uk/treatments/explore-all-treatments/treatment-add-ons/.

'Before embryo transfer, the glue is added to the solution in the dish containing the embryo': Treatment add-ons, HFEA [Online] Available from: https://www.hfea.gov.uk/treatments/explore-all-treatments/treatment-add-ons/.

'as babies from fresh cycle IVF have been known to have a lower birth weight': Spijkers, S, Lens, JW, Schats, R, Lambalk, C (2017) Fresh and Frozen-Thawed Embryo Transfer Compared to Natural Conception: Differences in Perinatal Outcome. [Online] Available from: https://www.ncbi.nlm.nih.gov/pmc/articles/PMC5804845/

'in the US, around a quarter of IVF cycles now use this strategy': Wilson, C. (2019) Freezing embryos doesn't boost IVF success rate despite common use, *New Scientist*, 24 June 2019. [Online] Available from: https://www.newscientist.com/article/2207380-freezing-embryos-doesnt-boost-ivf-success-rate-despite-common-use/.

'experts aren't sure yet whether freeze-all cycles are more effective': Wilson, C. (2019) Freezing embryos doesn't boost IVF success rate despite common use, *New Scientist*, 24 June 2019. Available from: https://www.newscientist.com/article/2207380-freezing-embryos-doesnt-boost-ivf-success-rate-despite-common-use/.

'a large-scale clinical trial called E-Freeze is happening at the moment': E-Freeze, National Perinatal Epidemiology Unit: https://www.npeu.ox.ac.uk/e-freeze.

'A time-lapse imaging system can also apply software to help the embryologist': Treatment add-ons, HFEA. [Online] Available from: https://www.hfea.gov.uk/treatments/ explore-all-treatments/treatment-add-ons/; Armstrong, S. *et al* (2019) Time-lapse systems for embryo incubation and embryo assessment for couples undergoing in vitro fertilisation and intracytoplasmic sperm injection, Cochrane Database systematic review, published 29 May 2019.

'(PGS) is a technique that tests embryos to see if they have the normal number of chromosomes': Pre-implantation genetic screening (PGS), HFEA. [Online] Available from: https://www.hfea.gov.uk/treatments/embryo-testing-and-treatments-for-disease/ pre-implantation-genetic-screening-pgs/.

'The HFEA has given PGS both an amber and red light rating': Treatment add-ons, HFEA. [Online] Available from: https://www.hfea.gov.uk/treatments/explore-all-treatments/ treatment-add-ons/.

'technique involves selecting the best sperm for ICSI, based on how they look': Treatment add-ons, HFEA. [Online] Available from: https://www.hfea.gov.uk/treatments/ explore-all-treatments/treatment-add-ons/.

'it involves putting sperm in a solution of hyaluronic acid (HA)': Treatment add-ons, HFEA. [Online] Available from: https://www.hfea.gov.uk/treatments/explore-all-treatments/treatment-add-ons/.

'calcium ionophores can be added to the Petri dish containing the egg and sperm': Treatment add-ons, HFEA. [Online] Available from: https://www.hfea.gov.uk/ treatments/explore-all-treatments/treatment-add-ons/.

'Intrauterine culture involves the egg being fertilised and placed in a device inserted into the mother's uterus': Treatment add-ons, HFEA. [Online] Available from: https:// www.hfea.gov.uk/treatments/explore-all-treatments/treatment-add-ons/.

'natural killer (uNK) cells are a major part of the white blood cell population in the endometrium': Natural killer cell, ScienceDaily. [Online] Available from: https:// www.sciencedaily.com/terms/natural_killer_cell.htm; The role of natural killer cells in human fertility, Royal College of Obstetrics and Gynaecology, Scientific Paper No 53, December 2016. [Online] Available from:
https://www.rcog.org.uk/globalassets/documents/guidelines/scientific-impact-papers/ sip_53.pdf.

'HFEA has given reproductive immunology tests and treatment a red light rating': Treatment add-ons, HFEA: https://www.hfea.gov.uk/treatments/explore-all-treatments/treatment-add-ons/.

'Take the case of the clinics offering money-back schemes': Finance and refund packages, The Fertility Partnership: https://www.gcrm.co.uk/prices/finance-and-refund-packages/. Access Fertility: www.accessfertility.com

'the story where a couple won a cycle of IVF': IVF baby Scottish mum 'won' in contest is born, BBC News, 26 July 2019. [Online] Available from: https://www.bbc.co.uk/news/ uk-scotland-edinburgh-east-fife-49129812

'claim to improve their chances of having a healthy baby when there is currently insufficient evidence': Wise, J. (2019) Show patients evidence for treatment 'add-ons', fertility clinics are told, *BMJ* 2019;364:1226. [Online] Available from: https://www. bmj.com/content/364/bmj.l226.

'the HFEA Chair Sally Cheshire told *The Telegraph* in an interview in 2019': Donnelly, L. (2019) Older women being exploited by IVF clinics - when just two a year will achieve success after the age of 44, *The Telegraph*, 21 April 2019. [Online] Available from: https://www.telegraph.co.uk/news/2019/04/21/older-women-exploited-ivf-clinics-just-two-year-will-achieve/.

'What the clinics shouldn't be doing is trading on hope and vulnerability': Donnelly, L. (2019) Older women being exploited by IVF clinics - when just two a year will achieve success after the age of 44, *The Telegraph*, 21 April 2019. [Online] Available from: https://www.telegraph.co.uk/news/2019/04/21/older-women-exploited-ivf-clinics-just-two-year-will-achieve/.

'The HFEA has no influence overseas to help you if something goes wrong': Fertility treatment abroad, HFEA. [Online] Available from: https://www.hfea.gov.uk/treatments/explore-all-treatments/fertility-treatment-abroad/

'some clinics offer it to help with "family balancing"': Sumathi Reddy (2015) 'Family balancing': Selecting your baby's gender, *Wall Street Journal* Lunch Break with Tanya Rivero, 17 August 2015. Available from: https://www.youtube.com/watch?v=V4t4IfAyhD8.

'Before 2005, the law ensures that donors can remain anonymous': (2015) UK national sperm bank has just nine donors, *BBC News*, 1 September 2015. [Online] Available from: https://www.bbc.co.uk/news/health-34113080.

'unless they choose to have that anonymity removed': Remove your donor anonymity, HFEA. [Online] Available from: https://www.hfea.gov.uk/donation/donors/remove-your-donor-anonymity/.

## CHAPTER 4

'Every year, around 1750 babies are born in this country using donated eggs or sperm': Getting started: Your guide to fertility treatment, HFEA [Online] Available from: https://ifqlive.blob.core.windows.net/umbraco-website/2110/hfea_a5_getting_started_guide_2017_pdf_for_upload_tagged_rev-1.pdf.

'Indeed, donor eggs can dramatically improve the chances' [Online] Source: www.hfea.gov.uk/about-us/publications/research-and-data/fertility-treatment-2018-trends-and-figures/.

'various other lifestyle factors could influence how the baby's genes are expressed': Epigenetics: can IVF affect your baby's genes? Your IVF journey. [Online] Available from: www.yourivfjourney.com/epigenetics-can-ivf-affect-your-babys-genes/.

'we humans are 99.9 per cent identical in terms of our DNA': Genetics vs. Genomics Fact Sheet, National Human Genome Research Institute. [Online] Available from: https://www.genome.gov/about-genomics/fact-sheets/Genetics-vs-Genomics.

'imagine a DNA sequence as the text of an instruction manual on how to make a human body': Rettner, R. (2017) DNA: Definition, structure and discovery, Live Science, 9 December 2017. [Online] Available from: https://www.livescience.com/37247-dna.html; *50 Ideas you really need to know: Biology*, JV Chamary (Quercus, London, 2015).

'epigenetic marks a bit like if someone highlights parts of the text in different colours': Ennis, C. (2014) Epigenetics 101: a beginner's guide to explaining everything, *The*

*Guardian*, 25 April 2014. [Online] Available from: https://www.theguardian.com/science/occams-corner/2014/apr/25/epigenetics-beginners-guide-to-everything.

'after fertilisation the embryo will be transferred to your uterus in the usual way': Getting started: Your guide to fertility treatment, HFEA. [Online] Available from: https://ifqlive.blob.core.windows.net/umbraco-website/2110/hfea_a5_getting_started_guide_2017_pdf_for_upload_tagged_rev-1.pdf.

'some of the treatment fees involved in donation (as of 2020) at the Bristol Centre for Reproductive Medicine': https://www.fertilitybristol.com/faqs-costs/costs/.

'if the donor donated before 1 April 2005 their anonymity is protected': Affordable treatment with no hidden costs, BCRM: https://www.hfea.gov.uk/donation/donors/remove-your-donor-anonymity/.

'Donors can only find out from the HFEA the number, sex and year of birth of any children': Getting started: Your guide to fertility treatment, HFEA. [Online] Available from: https://ifqlive.blob.core.windows.net/umbraco-website/2110/hfea_a5_getting_started_guide_2017_pdf_for_upload_tagged_rev-1.pdf.

'Provided a couple is married or in a civil partnership at that date': Becoming the legal parents of your child, HFEA [Online] Available from: https://www.hfea.gov.uk/treatments/explore-all-treatments/becoming-the-legal-parents-of-your-child/.

'to make sure that they are fully aware of the implications': (2018) Code of Practice, HFEA. [Online] Available from: https://www.hfea.gov.uk/media/2565/hfea-draft-code-of-practice-9th-edition-consultation-version.pdf

'They can also donate eggs, sperm or embryos for use in research': HFEA Getting started: Your guide to fertility treatment. [Online] Available from: https://ifqlive.blob.core.windows.net/umbraco-website/2110/hfea_a5_getting_started_guide_2017_pdf_for_upload_tagged_rev-1.pdf.

'sperm donors can donate sperm for up to 10 families and be paid up to £35 per clinic visit': Sperm donors and the law – for donors, HFEA. [Online] Available from: https://www.hfea.gov.uk/donation/donors/donating-your-sperm/sperm-donation-and-the-law-for-donors/.

'donors are only anonymous if they donated before 2005': Remove your donor anonymity, HFEA. [Online] Available from: https://www.hfea.gov.uk/donation/donors/remove-your-donor-anonymity/.

'after the law changed the number of women treated with donated sperm fell': Batty, D. and agencies (2008) Fertility treatment drops following ban on anonymous sperm donation, *The Guardian*, 26 June 2008. [Online] Available from: https://www.theguardian.com/uk/2008/jun/26/women.health.

'you will have to undergo various tests to make sure you don't pass on any medical conditions': Donating your eggs, HFEA. [Online] Available from: https://www.hfea.gov.uk/donation/donors/donating-your-eggs/.

'Egg donors get up to £750 per cycle of donation': Donating your eggs, HFEA: https://www.hfea.gov.uk/donation/donors/donating-your-eggs/.

'Around 70 per cent of sperm donors and egg donors were white British': Trends in egg and sperm donation, HFEA. [Online] Available from: www.hfea.gov.uk/media/2808/trends-in-egg-and-sperm-donation-final.pdf.

'Olivia sourced the sperm from the European Sperm Bank': Packham, A. (2018) A shortage of sperm donors: The Brexist dilemma we didn't see coming, *Huffington Post*,

12 November 2018. [Online] Available from: https://www.huffingtonpost.co.uk/entry/british-men-reluctant-sperm-donors_uk_5bbdfc4ae4b01470d057984a.

'f all women accessing fertility treatment (fresh IVF and donor insemination) with donated gametes in 2013, 17 per cent had no registered partner': Fertility treatment 2014–2016 Trends and figures, HFEA [Online] Available from: www.hfea.gov.uk/media/2563/hfea-fertility-trends-and-figures-2017-v2.pdf.

'the donor will have to have consented to any subsequent embryo being used': Donating your embryos, HFEA. [Online] Available from: https://www.hfea.gov.uk/donation/donors/donating-your-embryos/

# CHAPTER 5

'In 2018, 38 per cent of all IVF cycles involved frozen embryos.' [Online] Available from: https://www.hfea.gov.uk/about-us/publications/research-and-data/fertility-treatment-2018-trends-and-figures/#mainpoints.

'clinics are cutting down on the number of embryos transferred in one go': Fertility treatment 2017, trends and figures, HFEA, published May 2019 [Online] Available from: https://www.hfea.gov.uk/media/2894/fertility-treatment-2017-trends-and-figures-may-2019.pdf.

'the cryoprotectants act like a sort of antifreeze': Behr, B. (2005) How do embryos survive the freezing process? *Scientific American*, 13 June 2005. [Online] Available from: https://www.scientificamerican.com/article/how-do-embryos-survive-th/; Embryo freezing, HFEA: https://www.hfea.gov.uk/treatments/fertility-preservation/embryo-freezing/.

'When a frozen embryo is transferred depends on your personal situation': HFEA Getting started: Your guide to fertility treatment. [Online] Available from: https://ifqlive.blob.core.windows.net/umbraco-website/2110/hfea_a5_getting_started_guide_2017_pdf_for_upload_tagged_rev-1.pdf.

'the length of time that a frozen embryo is stored doesn't affect the chances of getting pregnant': Getting started: Your guide to fertility treatment, HFEA. [Online] Available from: https://ifqlive.blob.core.windows.net/umbraco-website/2110/hfea_a5_getting_started_guide_2017_pdf_for_upload_tagged_rev-1.pdf.

'in special circumstances embryos can be stored for up to 55 years': Embryo freezing, HFEA [Online] Available from: https://www.hfea.gov.uk/treatments/fertility-preservation/embryo-freezing/.

'success rates for frozen cycles are slightly higher at 23 per cent': Fertility treatment 2017, trends and figures, HFEA, published May 2019 [Online] Available from: https://www.hfea.gov.uk/media/2894/fertility-treatment-2017-trends-and-figuresmay-2019.pdf.

'a partner (or a donor) can withdraw consent': Embryo freezing, HFEA. [Online] Available from: https://www.hfea.gov.uk/treatments/fertility-preservation/embryo-freezing/

'there are all sorts of other reasons you may want to freeze your eggs': Egg freezing, HFEA. [Online] Available from: https://www.hfea.gov.uk/treatments/fertility-preservation/egg-freezing/

'egg freezing increased by 240 per cent from 2013 to 2018.' [Online] Available from: https://www.hfea.gov.uk/about-us/publications/research-and-data/fertility-treatment-2018-trends-and-figures/#storage.

'only 19 per cent of IVF treatments using a patient's own frozen eggs were successful': Davis, N. (2018) Women need more realistic data on egg-freezing success, say experts, *The Guardian*, 8 August 2018. [Online] Available from: https://www.theguardian.com/science/2018/aug/08/women-need-more-realistic-data-on-egg-freezing-success-say-experts.

'research has suggested that using frozen eggs leads to higher rates of miscarriage': Egg freezing, HFEA. [Online] Available from: https://www.hfea.gov.uk/treatments/fertility-preservation/egg-freezing/.

'the best time to freeze eggs is in your early 20s': Davis, N. (2018) Women need more realistic data on egg-freezing success, say experts, *The Guardian*, 8 August 2018. [Online] Available from: https://www.theguardian.com/science/2018/aug/08/women-need-more-realistic-data-on-egg-freezing-success-say-experts.

'if a woman freezes her eggs before she turns 35, the chances of success are higher than conceiving naturally as she gets older': Egg freezing in fertility treatment, Trends and figures: 2010–2016, HFEA. [Online] Available from: https://www.hfea.gov.uk/about-us/news-and-press-releases/2018-news-and-press-releases/press-release-age-is-the-key-factor-for-egg-freezing-success-says-new-hfea-report-as-overall-treatment-numbers-remain-low/.

'experts felt that doctors should initiate discussion about fertility decline': Yu, L. *et al* (2016) Knowledge, attitudes, and intentions toward fertility awareness and oocyte cryopreservation among obstetrics and gynecology resident physicians, *Human Reproduction* 31(2), 403–411.

'if you've got a medical condition requiring treatment that will affect your fertility': Egg freezing, HFEA: https://www.hfea.gov.uk/treatments/fertility-preservation/egg-freezing/.

'In France, egg freezing is currently only allowed in cases where a patient is likely to become infertile': Collins, Y. (2019) France considers allowing IVF for single and lesbian women, BioNews, 17 June 2019. [Online] Available from: https://www.bionews.org.uk/page_143371; http://www.rfi.fr/en/france/20191128-french-fertility-doctors-bend-law-allow-women-freeze-eggs-ivf-pregnancy-illegal-vote and https://www.politico.eu/article/france-warms-up-to-egg-freezing/.

'worth discussing this option in depth with consultants and other professionals treating you for medical conditions': Getting started: Your guide to fertility treatment, HFEA. [Online] Available from: https://ifqlive.blob.core.windows.net/umbraco-website/2110/hfea_a5_getting_started_guide_2017_pdf_for_upload_tagged_rev-1.pdf.

'If you're about to go through gender reassignment treatment': Information for trans and non-binary people seeking fertility treatment, HFEA. [Online] Available from: https://www.hfea.gov.uk/treatments/fertility-preservation/information-for-trans-and-non-binary-people-seeking-fertility-treatment/.

'research suggests that long-term sperm freezing makes little difference to live birth rates': (2019) Storing sperm in a freezer for a decade hardly affects birth rates, *New Scientist*, 24 June 2019. [Online] Available from: https://www.newscientist.com/article/2207447-storing-sperm-in-a-freezer-for-a-decade-hardly-affects-birth-rates/.

'Freezing your sperm could be useful if...': Sperm freezing, HFEA. [Online] Available from: https://www.hfea.gov.uk/treatments/fertility-preservation/sperm-freezing/.

'This involves freezing a small piece of tissue from a testicle': HFEA Getting started: Your guide to fertility treatment. [Online] Available from: https://ifqlive.blob.core. windows.net/umbraco-website/2110/hfea_a5_getting_started_guide_2017_pdf_for_ upload_tagged_rev-1.pdf.

'in 2019, a group of women brought the UK's first legal challenge to the 10-year limit on preserving frozen eggs': Henriques, M. (2019) First legal challenge to 10-year limit on egg freezing, BioNews, 18 March 2019. [Online] Available from: https://www.bionews. org.uk/page_142043.

'this is a matter for parliament to change legislation': Egg freezing in fertility treatment, Trends and figures: 2010–2016, HFEA. [Online] Available from: https://www.hfea.gov.uk/ media/2656/egg-freezing-in-fertility-treatment-trends-and-figures-2010-2016-final.pdf.

'case where a dead man's testes were removed and put into': Davey, M. (2016) Parents likely to block girlfriend's attempt to access sperm from dead son, The Guardian, 1 June 2016. [Online] Available from:
www.theguardian.com/science/2016/jun/01/parents-likely-to-block-girlfriends-attempt-to-access-sperm-from-dead-son.

'French authorities allowed a woman to take the sperm her husband froze before he died to Spain for IVF': Credi, B. (2016) French judges authorise use of dead husband's sperm for IVF, West, 6 January 2016. [Online] Available from: https://www.west-info. eu/french-judges-authorise-use-of-dead-husbands-sperm-for-ivf/.

'Both were conceived through IVF, using sperm harvested when Stephen was in a coma': (1997) Widow allowed dead husband's baby, BBC News, 6 February 1997. [Online] Available from: http://news.bbc.co.uk/onthisday/hi/dates/stories/february/6/ newsid_2536000/2536119.stm;

Lambert, V. (2017) Exclusive: Diane Blood on family life 20 years after she won the right to use her dead husband's sperm, The Telegraph, 10 February 2017. [Online] Available from: https://www.telegraph.co.uk/women/family/exclusive-diane-blood-family-life-20-years-won-right-use-dead/.

## CHAPTER 6

'The average live birth rate for each embryo transferred for women of any age is 22 per cent': Fertility trends explained, Fertility treatment 2017: trends and figures report, HFEA, published May 2019. [Online] Available from: https://www.hfea.gov.uk/about-us/publications/research-and-data/fertility-trends-explained/

'the chance of getting pregnant from future treatment was 10 per cent higher for women who had previously had a miscarriage': (2017) Hope for couples suffering IVF miscarriages, University of Aberdeen News, 20 September 2017. [Online] Available from https://www.abdn.ac.uk/news/11145/.

'Contact your clinic if you're experiencing pain in your abdomen and bleeding that looks unusual': Ectopic pregnancy: symptoms, NHS: https://www.nhs.uk/conditions/ ectopic-pregnancy/symptoms/

'no escaping the fact that these are no mere specks of blood, but the womb lining leaving my body': Periods and fertility in the menstrual cycle, NHS: https://www.nhs.uk/Livewell/ menstrualcycle/Pages/Whatisthemenstrualcycle.aspx.

'If IVF hasn't worked for you, you might want to consider other options, such as surrogacy or adoption.': https://www.hfea.gov.uk/treatments/explore-all-treatments/surrogacy/ https://www.adoptionuk.org/about-modern-adoption

'A directory of accredited private therapists': IVF: support, NHS: https://www.nhs.uk/conditions/ivf/support/; Getting emotional support, HFEA. [Online] Available from: https://www.hfea.gov.uk/treatments/explore-all-treatments/getting-emotional-support/.


## CHAPTER 7

Sources: HFEA Fertility Treatment 2017: Trends and Figures report published in 2019. HFEA Fertility Treatment 2018: Trends and Figures report published in 2020.

'the procedure was carried out simply to help an infertile couple who had already been through four cycles of IVF': Gallagher, J. (2019) 'Three-person' baby boy born in Greece, BBC News, 11 April 2019. [Online] Available from: https://www.bbc.co.uk/news/health-47889387.

'only people with a very high risk of passing a serious mitochondrial disease on to their children are eligible for treatment': Mitochondrial donation treatment, HFEA. [Online] Available from: https://www.hfea.gov.uk/treatments/embryo-testing-and-treatments-for-disease/mitochondrial-donation-treatment/.

'the uterus of a 45-year-old donor…was transplanted into a 32-year-old woman': Ejzenberg, D. et al (2018) Livebirth after uterus transplantation from a deceased donor in a recipient with uterine infertility, The Lancet, 392(10165), pp. 2697–2704. [Online] Available from: https://www.thelancet.com/journals/lancet/article/PIIS0140-67361831766-5/fulltext.

'could actually detect the embryo's genetic make-up better than the traditional biopsy method': Kuznyetsov, V. et al (2018) Evaluation of a novel non-invasive preimplantation genetic screening approach, PLoS One 13(5): e0197262. https://www.ncbi.nlm.nih.gov/pmc/articles/PMC5944986/; Siristatidis, C.S. et al (2018) Metabolomics for improving pregnancy outcomes, Cochrane, 16 March 2018. [Online] Available from: https://www.cochrane.org/CD011872/MENSTR_metabolomics-improving-pregnancy-outcomes; Hernandez, D. (2019) New noninvasive genetic tests for IVF embryos are in development, The Wall Street Journal, 24 June 2019. [Online] Available from: https://www.wsj.com/articles/new-noninvasive-genetic-tests-for-ivf-embryos-are-in-development-11561402801.

'the success of an embryo implanting in the endometrium is influenced by the presence of microbes': https://www.ncbi.nlm.nih.gov/pubmed/31119299; https://www.rbmojournal.com/article/S1472-6483(17)30187-6/pdf; https://www.ncbi.nlm.nih.gov/pmc/articles/PMC6910115/

'more research is needed to understand how this impacts fertility': García-Velasco, J.A. et al (2017) What fertility specialists should know about the vaginal microbiome: a review, Reproductive BioMedicine Online 35(1), pp. 103–112; Koedooder, R. et al (2019) The vaginal microbiome as a predictor for outcome of in vitro fertilization with or without intracytoplasmic sperm injection: a prospective study, Human Reproduction 34(6), pp. 1042–1054.

'providing info on things such as predicting ovulation and tracking hormone levels': Ducharme, J. How artificial intelligence could change the fertility world, Time [Online]

Available from: https://time.com/collection/life-reinvented/5492063/artificial-intelligence-fertility/.

'start-up that uses machine learning to crunch the data from patients' lab tests': https://www.forbes.com/sites/zarastone/2019/03/19/ivf-and-ai-how-univfy-startup-uses-machine-learning-to-make-fertility-smarter/#2a9a118866ff

'Future Fertility has created the egg-scoring algorithm Violet': Molteni, M. (2019) Women may soon start using AI to tell good eggs from bad, *Wired*, 30 April 2019. [Online] Available from: https://www.wired.com/story/women-may-soon-start-using-ai-to-tell-good-eggs-from-bad/.

'researchers at Weill Cornell Medicine in the US': (2019) Artificial intelligence approach optimizes embryo selection for IVF, Weill Cornell Medicine News, 4 April 2019. [Online] Available from: https://news.weill.cornell.edu/news/2019/04/artificial-intelligence-approach-optimizes-embryo-selection-for-ivf.

'a company called Life Whisperer has developed a similar AI': (2018) AI tool to predict IVF success moves closer to commercialisation, Life Whisperer (from *The Lead*, 9 August 2018). [Online] Available from: https://www.lifewhisperer.co/ai-tool-to-predict-ivf-success-moves-closer-to-commercialisation/ .

'prior to implantation, the blastocyst is actively sensing its environment': Aljahdali, A.R. (2017) Effect of *in vitro* fertilisation (IVF) and embryo culture duration on mouse development and postnatal health, PhD thesis. [Online] Available from: https://eprints.soton.ac.uk/413958/1/PhD_Final_Thesis_Anan_Aljahdali_9_June_2017. pdf.

'the gene editing technique known as "CRISPR Cas-9" has been revolutionising the world of genetics': Le Page, M. and Klein, A. (2018) World's first gene-edited babies announced by a scientist in China, *New Scientist*, 26 November 2018. [Online] Available from: https://www.newscientist.com/article/2186504-worlds-first-gene-edited-babies-announced-by-a-scientist-in-china/.

'did not actually produce the desired result and could have caused unwanted or 'off-target' mutations': Le Page, M. and Klein, A. (2018) World's first gene-edited babies announced by a scientist in China, *New Scientist*, 26 November 2018. [Online] Available from: https://www.newscientist.com/article/2186504-worlds-first-gene-edited-babies-announced-by-a-scientist-in-china/; Cyranoski, D. (2019) China to tighten rules on gene editing in humans, *Nature*, 6 March 2019. [Online] Available from: https://www.nature.com/articles/d41586-019-00773-y; Cohen, J. (2019) The untold story of the 'circle of trust' behind the world's first gene-edited babies, *Science*, 1 August 2019. [Online] Available from: https://www.sciencemag.org/news/2019/08/untold-story-circle-trust-behind-world-s-first-gene-edited-babies; Agence France-Presse (2019) China gene-edited baby experiment 'may have created unintended mutations', *The Guardian*, 4 December 2019. [Online] Available from: https://www.theguardian.com/science/2019/dec/04/china-gene-edited-baby-experiment-may-have-created-unintended-mutations; Seidel, G. (2018) How a scientist says he made a gene-edited baby – and what health worries may ensue, The Conversation, 29 November 2018. [Online] Available from: https://theconversation.com/how-a-scientist-says-he-made-a-gene-edited-baby-and-what-health-worries-may-ensue-107764.

'there have been calls for a rapid review of the ethics and much tougher penalties for breaking the rules': Ledford, H. (2019) CRISPR babies: when will the world be read?

*Nature*, 24 June 2019. [Online] Available from: https://www.nature.com/articles/ d41586-019-01906-z; Berg, J. (2017) Editing human embryos with CRISPR is moving ahead – now's the time to work out the ethics, The Conversation, 28 July 2017. [Online] Available from: http://theconversation.com/editing-human-embryos-with-crispr-is-moving-ahead-nows-the-time-to-work-out-the-ethics-81732; (2017) Take stock of research ethics in human genome editing, *Nature* 549, p. 307. [Online] Available from: https://www.nature.com/news/take-stock-of-research-ethics-in-human-genome-editing-1.22632.

'the ethics body did highlight the importance of research into the safety of such gene editing':

Sample, I. (2018) Genetically modified babies given go ahead by UK ethics body, *The Guardian*, 17 July 2018. [Online] Available from: https://www.theguardian.com/ science/2018/jul/17/genetically-modified-babies-given-go-ahead-by-uk-ethics-body; Janssens, A.C.J.W. (2018) Those designer babies everyone is freaking out about – it's not likely to happen, The Conversation, 10 December 2018. [Online] Available from: http://theconversation.com/those-designer-babies-everyone-is-freaking-out-about-its-not-likely-to-happen-103079.

'selecting traits brought about by multiple genes ... is actually very complicated': Janssens, A.C.J.W. (2018) Those designer babies everyone is freaking out about – it's not likely to happen, The Conversation, 10 December 2018. [Online] Available from: https:// theconversation.com/those-designer-babies-everyone-is-freaking-out-about-its-not-likely-to-happen-103079.

'the computer simulations showed that any advantage was actually minimal': (2019) Simulations suggest embryo selection based on traits like height or IQ is still far off, EurekAlert!, 21 November 2019. [Online] Available from: https://www.eurekalert.org/ pub_releases/2019-11/cp-sse111419.php.

'as well as identify embryos that are likely to have below average intelligence': Regelado, A. (2019) The world's first Gattaca baby tests are finally here, Technology Review, 8 November 2019. [Online] Available from: https://www.technologyreview. com/s/614690/polygenic-score-ivf-embryo-dna-tests-genomic-prediction-gattaca/; Wilson, C. (2018) A new test can predict IVF embryos' risk of having a low IQ, *New Scientist*, 15 November 2018. [Online] Available from: https://www.newscientist. com/article/mg24032041-900-exclusive-a-new-test-can-predict-ivf-embryos-risk-of-having-a-low-iq/; (2018) New techniques may soon make designer babies a reality – are we ready? *New Scientist*, 15 November 2018. [Online] Available from: https:// www.newscientist.com/article/mg24032041-800-new-techniques-may-soon-make-designer-babies-a-reality-are-we-ready/; Ball, P. (2018) Super-smart designer babies could be on offer soon. But is that ethical? *The Guardian*, 19 November 2018. [Online] Available from: https://www.theguardian.com/commentisfree/2018/nov/19/designer-babies-ethical-genetic-selection-intelligence.

'where genetic selection ensures children possess the best hereditary traits of their parents': Regelado, A. (2019) The world's first Gattaca baby tests are finally here, Technology Review, 8 November 2019. [Online] Available from: https://www.technologyreview. com/s/614690/polygenic-score-ivf-embryo-dna-tests-genomic-prediction-gattaca/.

'Scientists in Japan have managed this in mice and created primordial germ cells': Ball, P. (2018) Reproduction revolution: how our skin cells might be turned into sperm and eggs, *The Guardian*, 14 October 2018. [Online] Available from: https://www.

theguardian.com/science/2018/oct/14/scientists-create-sperm-eggs-using-skin-cells-fertility-ethical-questions.

'After four days, the cells had formed a structure resembling a mouse embryo': Harrison, S. and Recher, G. (2017) Scientists at the University of Cambridge have managed to create a structure resembling a mouse embryo in culture, using two types of stem cells – the body's 'master cells' – and a 3D scaffold on which they can grow, University of Cambridge research news, 2 March 2017. [Online] Available from: https://www.cam.ac.uk/research/news/scientists-create-artificial-mouse-embryo-from-stem-cells-for-first-time.

'scientists in the US have used human stem cells to make structures that mimic early embryos': Cyranoski, D. (2019) Embryo-like structures created from human stem cells, Nature, 11 September 2019. [Online] Available from: https://www.nature.com/articles/d41586-019-02654-w.

'Fertility experts also see the potential for use in IVF for patients who aren't able to carry for a full pregnancy': Romanis, E.C. (2019) We need to talk about the artificial womb, BioNews, 14 October 2019. [Online] Available from: https://www.bionews.org.uk/page_145577; https://gizmodo.com/artificial-wombs-are-getting-better-and-better-1833639606.

'[PGD] is already being used for sex selection in the US to help with "family balancing"': Sumathi Reddy (2015) 'Family balancing': Selecting your baby's gender, Wall Street Journal Lunch Break with Tanya Rivero, 17 August 2015. Available from: https://www.youtube.com/watch?v=V4t4IfAyhD8.

'sperm can be picked to fertilise the egg so that offspring are male (XY) or female (XX)': Davis, N. (2019) Sperm separation method may allow sex selection in IVF, The Guardian, 13 August 2019. [Online] Available from: https://www.theguardian.com/science/2019/aug/13/sperm-separation-method-may-allow-gender-selection-in-ivf.

'scientists managed to remove the extra sex chromosome in mice to produce fertile offspring': The Francis Crick Institute (2017) New technique overcomes genetic cause of infertility, ScienceDaily, 17 August 2017. Available from: https://www.sciencedaily.com/releases/2017/08/170817141800.htm.

'Cutting the ovaries into pieces was found to slow down growth, meaning that egg supply was conserved': Conger, K. (2013) Technique induces egg growth in infertile women, and one gives birth, Stanford Medicine News Center, 30 September 2013. Available from: http://med.stanford.edu/news/all-news/2013/09/technique-induces-egg-growth-in-infertile-women-and-one-gives-birth.html; Kawamura, K. et al (2016) Activation of dormant follicles: a new treatment for premature ovarian failure? Current Opinion in Obstetrics and Gynecology 28(3), pp. 217–222.

'the researchers managed to restart periods in around 30 women between the ages of 46 and 49': Hamzelou, J. (2016) Menopause reversal restores periods and produces fertile eggs, New Scientist, 20 July 2016. [Online] Available from: https://www.newscientist.com/article/mg23130833-100-menopause-reversal-restores-periods-and-produces-fertile-eggs/.

'a fresh set of 'batteries' transferred from more youthful ovarian cells': Connor S. (2016) The next IVF revolution: Older women more likely to have babies with new technique set to trial in UK this year, Independent, 25 January 2016. [Online] Available from:

https://www.independent.co.uk/news/science/ivf-procedure-that-makes-older-eggs-young-again-could-come-to-uk-a6831736.html.

'meaning it could theoretically be possible to extend a women's fertility by up to six years': Fuller-Wright, L. (2018) Fertility breakthrough: New research could extend egg health with age, Princeton University Office of Communications, 22 February 2018. [Online] Available from: https://www.princeton.edu/news/2018/02/22/fertility-breakthrough-new-research-could-extend-egg-health-age.

'a Vatican official strongly disapproved of one of the IVF pioneers receiving a Nobel Prize': https://www.bbc.co.uk/news/health-11472753

# Acknowledgements

E ach time I look at our two girls, I marvel at the complexity of their bodies and the fact that they were once just a sperm and an egg. I'm not a religious person, but conception, birth and the development of any creature truly astounds me. The miracle of life.

I'm eternally grateful to all the researchers around the world who have developed the science of IVF. I'm also hugely grateful to Dr Chandra Kailasam for your expertise, which enabled us to have our two girls, and all the talented staff at the Bristol Centre for Reproductive Medicine (BCRM) at Southmead Hospital in Bristol.

Thank you also to all the patients who gave their time to be interviewed for this book, and all the experts: Nina Barnsley, Director of the Donor Conception Network (DCN); Prof. Jacky Boivin from the University of Cardiff; Dr Cesar Diaz-Garcia, Medical Director IVI London; Dr Chandra Kailasam, Consultant in Reproductive Medicine at the London Women's Clinic; Prof. Edzard Ernst, Emeritus Professor at the University of Exeter; Natalie Gamble, fertility lawyer, NGA Law; Wendy Martin, Fertility Therapist at the Bristol Centre for Reproductive Medicine (BCRM); Prof. Geeta Nargund, Medical Director, CREATE Fertility; Prof. Robert Norman from the University of Adelaide; Prof. Allan Pacey from the University of Sheffield; Barbara Scott, Chair of the Association of Reproductive Reflexologists; Prof. Richard Sharpe from the University of Edinburgh; and Paul Wilson, BCRM Head of Embryology and Andrology. Thank you also to the HFEA for your work confirming stats and providing sources.

A special thank you to Dr Valentine Akande, Dr Chandra Kailasam and Dr JV Chamary for your help and guidance with this book.

And, finally, thank you to my family – particularly my amazing sister, Tamara, who supported us through the whole IVF process and is now the most incredible aunt, adored by her nieces. And to my husband, Max – you're wonderful. Thank you for going on this IVF journey with me, surviving the whirlwind of bringing up our girls, and also supporting me to write this book. Without your support (and your sperm!), none of this would have been possible.

# Index